TWENTIETH CENTURY STUDIES

edited by

Donald Tyerman

THE NEW DIMENSIONS OF MEDICINE

Twentieth Century Studies

THE NEW DIMENSIONS
OF MEDICINE

by

ALAN NORTON

D.M., D.P.M.

HODDER AND STOUGHTON

Printed in Great Britain for Hodder and Stoughton Limited, St. Paul's House, Warwick
Lane, London, E.C.4, by C. Tinling & Co. Ltd., Liverpool, London and Prescot

Editor's Preface

After the parson the doctor. This is the second book in the series of Twentieth Century Studies. The first—*Religion and Change*, by David Edwards—looked at the role of religious belief in the secularised society of this century. *The New Dimensions of Medicine*, by Alan Norton, looks at the tremendous impact of scientific advance, and of the century's great social changes, on medical theory, practice and organisation, on the concepts of health and disease, and on the prospects of life and death. From their very different viewpoints both books till the same teeming field of human existence in this century of technological and political transformation and turbulence. Both treat of the distinctive hopes and fears and expectations of our times. Both bear out Alexis de Tocqueville's description—"Not a history, not a series of philosophical observations; but a mixture of the two" —which we have taken as the rubric for all these Studies.

The purpose of these books, as it will be of all the succeeding volumes in the series, is not simply to tell the story of the century's events in each separate field of inquiry. Nor is it simply to set out the development of ideas in each separate field of thought. It is, essentially, to marry the events with the issues, the narrative with the notions, the history with the philosophical observations, as de Tocqueville did. It is to show the interplay between what men have thought, and thought out, and what they have done, or tried to do. Each Study takes as its province a characteristic change in twentieth century thought and practice. All are written, and edited, with this common and, I believe, distinctive purpose in mind. But each is the separate and independent responsibility of its author.

Nobody who even glances at the world today, whether at the life of individuals in modern communities or at the cheek-by-jowl problems of poverty and affluence, at the population explosion and the technological revolution, or at the tensions that hold peace always in the balance, can doubt the central significance of the new dimensions of medicine in the twentieth century. Nobody who reads Alan Norton's clear and precise recension, stage by stage, of what the doctors and the scientists have been able to do so far and, even more, what they have still to do, can believe that there are any final solutions, any absolute progress, as the new opportunities are overtaken by the new problems of new ways of living, while old problems across much of the world stay unresolved.

Spectacular progress there has been. Alan Norton has charted it, fully and feelingly but soberly, from his special standpoint as a busily expert psychiatrist with the widest medical experience and scientific interest. But he spells out equally plainly the new riddles, ethical and humane as well as scientific and social, political and economic, that stem from man's new-found capacity to control his bodily and mental fate.

"Yet all experience is an arch wherethro'
Gleams that untravell'd world, whose margin fades
For ever and for ever when I move."

Donald Tyerman

Preface

A book on this subject could more easily have been written by a syndicate of experts. If it had, each author would certainly have explored his subject more penetratingly and accurately than I have done. But the medical editor would not have had an easy task. Having chosen his topics and his experts would he have been able to avoid overlapping and could he have kept all his team dancing to his themes? Or would they all have performed individual variations? Unless he was very skilful and lucky his book would have lacked the synoptic view. And a synoptic view is necessary for the book to show the interaction between medicine and its twentieth century setting.

If there was to be a single author need a psychiatrist these days apologise for having attempted the task? I hope not. Psychiatry is influenced by and itself influences many of the matters dealt with in the book. Its use of the new drugs, its intimate involvement in community and preventive medicine, and its close relation to geriatrics are prime examples. Its role as an alternative to older methods of dealing with delinquent behaviour and its tentative efforts to contain so many of the new diseases ensure that psychiatry already has a central place in twentieth century medicine. Psychiatry, too, is one of the few specialties in which, since the war, Britain has led the world.

I have to acknowledge a great deal of help from friends and colleagues. This, I hope, has kept me on the right lines and avoided gross errors. I should not like any of them to be held responsible for anything I have said, for as often as not they saw only an earlier version and not the final manuscript. I am grateful to my colleagues at Bexley and Lewisham Hospitals: D. Bannister, A. E. R. Buckle, C. A. Holman, D. M. Leiberman, Mary McMillan, T. M. L. Price, J. S. Staffurth and J. H. P. Willis. Others who have helped include C. Cherry of the University of Kent at Canterbury, Marjorie Deane of *The Economist*, H. E. Hobbs of the Royal Free Hospital, and A. W. Tranter, Deputy Medical Officer of Health for Lewisham. I am particularly grateful to my colleague Andrew Smith, who read most of the original manuscript and whose criticism was most welcome and almost always heeded.

I should like to record my thanks to several members of the staff of the Statistics Unit of the General Register Office and I am happy to acknowledge the Registrar General's permission to reproduce figures from his publications in tables and in charts. These charts were kindly drawn for me by Richard Natkiel of *The Economist*.

I owe a big debt to the editor of the series, Donald Tyerman, whose help in giving coherence to my ill-organised thoughts has been invaluable, and to the publishers, particularly Christopher Stobart, not only for their tolerance but also for suggestions and criticisms that were always helpful and sometimes crucial. My wife wrote Chapter 12 and has also overseen my grammar and punctuation.

July 1968

Contents

CHAPTER ONE

The Changing World of Medicine

To pin down medicine[1] at a moment in time, to analyse it, to identify the broad trends of change during this century, their sources, their influence, and where they are leading to; to chart the feed-back, the powerful effects that changes in medicine in turn have had on society and on the life and outlook of individuals—these are the chief aims of this book and a daunting enough task. But the static anatomical analogy, the metaphor of dissection, makes the task seem simpler than in fact it is, for those abstractions "medicine" and "diseases" have no meaning when divorced from the people who practise it and those who suffer from them. These people, we ourselves, patients and doctors, have not remained miraculously unchanged while "the science and art" of medicine have advanced in this century but have inevitably been moulded by the seminal ideas, and the social and educational changes that have pervaded our lifetime, and particularly by the scientific and technical revolution. The practice of medicine has been transformed in advanced societies by a network of forces. These range—to give a few examples—from the spread of literacy to the ideas of Freud, and from an increasing economic security to a decline in religious observance. They include the trend to social equality and, not least in importance, a revolution in the ease of communication in every sense of that word.

In the practice of medicine itself there have been far-reaching changes in the meaning of the basic terms in the equation. A *doctor*, for example, may work for a drug firm and never see a patient, or he may be an experimental scientist; a *patient* may be a well person undergoing a screening test, or he may have changed his label from that of "criminal" or "difficult child"; the *relationship* between patient and doctor can range from the exceedingly intense in psychoanalysis to the non-existent in large-scale preventive medicine. *Disease* now includes not only childhood behaviour disorders and, say, a need for

---

[1] "The science and art concerned with the cure, alleviation and prevention of disease . . ." *The Shorter Oxford English Dictionary*. (Clarendon Press. Oxford, 1944. 3rd. ed.).

contraceptive advice, but also a host of conditions produced by efforts at treatment—the iatrogenic diseases. The *context* of medicine, both physical and financial, has perhaps changed most of all with the development on the one hand of health centres, specialised clinics and industrial health services, and on the other of compulsory health insurance and national health services in most advanced countries.

These five elements in the transaction are as closely inter-related as the components of a mobile, so that any change in one produced by an external influence—say, the growth of medical journalism in mass media, or an increasing abuse of "hard" drugs by the young— causes a disturbance in the system till a new balance is struck. But time and again the disturbance spreads outside medicine to invade the social and economic field. Should addiction belong to medicine or is it to be dealt with by the law and the police? How many kidney machines can a country properly afford? Should cigarette- smoking be banned? Are changes in the law required to make it easier for organs to be obtained for transplantation? This disconcert- ing tendency of medicine to throw the ball back to society and by its very progress to create further dilemmas is a specifically twentieth century phenomenon. Most of the chapters in this book contain examples, and society has yet to find ways round many of them.

The challenge to society from the new medicine originates over- whelmingly from the invasion of medicine by science, and today, in that medicine is a science, it is an applied science. In relation to other sciences and to society medicine is a passively reacting system—the image of the mobile is apt. Scientific medicine has taken as much from science as it has given back to the world; but this is not to decry its gifts, which have been substantial.

There was a time, not very long ago, when medicine was not so passive, when the great advances came from people actually practis- ing the art. Diseases were recognised, classified, and named after their discoverers. Bright, Addison, Sydenham, Charcot and Graves were practitioners. This era continued into the present century— Cushing, for example—but since then medicine has been increasingly dependent for its advances on discoveries elsewhere. Nowadays, the pioneers are seldom practising doctors, even if, like Banting, Fleming, Florey and Burnet, they may incidentally be medically qualified. There are exceptions, of course—Freud, the chief among them, and Pavlov, the father of behaviour therapy. But within medicine nowa- days the important people are either administrators or technical innovators. The important ideas come from outside; from people such as Pincus, who pioneered the Pill, and Medawar with his studies in immunology. The picture, then, of modern medicine is of a sensitive system reacting to changes outside itself—applying lasers, for example, adapting teaching machines, choosing the most suitable plastic for a hundred uses, automating its laboratory processes, utilising the one gene=one enzyme concept, or deriving behaviour therapy from learning theory.

Doctors may have ceased to be innovators, but together with their patients they are children of their own age. Each great secular change has had profound effects on them and often on their relationship. To take five examples—others will be discussed later:

a. The spread of literacy and education—this has narrowed the intellectual gap between the doctor and most of his patients. Coupled with the vastly increased amount of information available it has made patients more knowledgeable, more critical. They need explanations. Blind faith and an autocratic manner are out of place as elements of the doctor-patient relationship today.

b. The trend towards massive organisations—in politics, economics and industry—has not left medicine untouched. Even if the basic person-to-person encounter has remained relatively unaltered, the spread of group practice has meant that quite often a patient cannot see the doctor of his choice. The context in which medicine is practised is increasingly determined by central control. The state in Britain owns nearly all the hospitals and for reasons of efficiency and economy these are becoming more standard in design and equipment. For those who work in hospitals the state is a near-monopoly employer. The doctors, too, are more tightly organised to improve their position in negotiations; even patients, conscious of their increasing power as consumers, are starting to form organisations to protect their interests.

c. New and pervasive psychological theories—widely accepted in medicine and by laymen—have given doctors new insight into the emotional origin of many patients' symptoms and, furthermore, have encouraged patients to seek medical aid when they would not previously have done so. They have thrown light on the nature of the relationship itself and have widened the scope of medicine because, being determinist, they have eroded age-old concepts of sin, crime, and personal responsibility.

d. The increasing influence of mass media of communication—the press, the radio and television with their voracious appetite for dramatic events and controversial issues have seized on medicine's technical advances. Public debates have been held on matters of intense public interest such as the moral aspects of abortion on social grounds and of contraception for the unmarried, or the serious and complex ethical problems of kidney and heart transplantation, before these matters have been thrashed out within the profession. A slow-moving and conservative profession, caught unawares by the speed of technical advance, has often seemed in disarray. For this reason, and there are others, doctors have lost some of their authority.

e. Increased permissiveness—this trend in morality,[1] similar in many ways to Taylor's[2] matristic swing (which he contrasts with the patristic-authoritarian), is a convenient term to describe many of the mid-twentieth century attitudes. It implies a diminished respect for authority figures and for the trappings of authority in dress and in ceremony; an increased freedom in the discussion of sexual matters and a tolerance of some forms of sexual behaviour previously frowned on; a changed attitude to the upbringing of children; a tendency to regard a larger slice of deviant behaviour as meriting treatment rather than punishment; and a greater tolerance of minority opinion. Much of the growth of psychiatry stems from this source, especially the demand for child psychiatry and for "treatment" for criminal behaviour and unusual sexual urges. But the demand for widened grounds for termination of pregnancy and for help with contraception, the increased tolerance of mental abnormality in the community's midst, and the present determination to leave the problem of drug addiction very largely in medical hands—all have their roots in this very twentieth century characteristic.

The Plan of the Book

Pride of place must be given, in any account of the influences moulding medicine in this century, to its invasion by science. This, more than anything else, would make the practice of medicine unrecognisable now to anyone from an earlier age.

The blossoming of knowledge and the multiplication of technique are discussed in Chapter 2: the cascade of drugs in Chapter 3. On *doctors* the effects of this revolution have been immense. They have included a necessity to specialise that has resulted in the near-fragmentation of the profession. Some specialties have developed concepts and a language all their own, which make communication even within medicine increasingly difficult. In addition, the secular reverence that society accords to the expert has intensified the rift between specialist and generalist and has made a satisfying career

[1] Whiteley, C. H. and W. M. *The Permissive Morality*. (Methuen. London, 1964).
[2] Taylor, Gordon Rattray. *Sex in History*. (Thames and Hudson. London, 1953).

for the general doctor, whom all societies probably need, difficult to attain. The sprouting of science within medicine, moreover, has led to the development of a new branch—experimental medicine—in which despite its virtues there are dangers within one man of the doctor-scientist conflicting with the doctor-physician. Drugs and new techniques have invested him with a power he never had before, but a power to harm as well as to heal—the new iatrogenic diseases are a witness to this. In fact, science in controlling old *diseases* has given birth to new ones.

As a side-effect (a word increasingly used nowadays) the late twentieth century doctor finds himself in an unfamiliar situation. He is the channel through which all "ethical" drugs are sold, the retailer and therefore the focus on which a rich new industry that he has helped to create concentrates its modern and sophisticated salesmanship.

For the *patient* the benefits have been immense. Modern scientific medicine has joined with economic advance and the egalitarian trend to produce in the people of Western countries an access of self-confidence. Political tyranny there ended twenty years ago, grave economic disruption longer ago still; now the horrid lurking insecurity of infectious disease that can strike people down in childhood or in their prime has evaporated. No wonder that patients vociferously demand access to vaunted science and technology, often brushing the generalist unwisely aside, to his dismay. It is ironic that this confidence in control of day-to-day matters should have coincided with the looming possibility of ultimate cosmic catastrophe.

The *relationship* between doctor and patient has also changed under the impact of science. In part the transaction has become to some slight extent commercial and the personalities of the two need have little contact. A prescription for the right pill may be all that is required or else a simple investigation clinches the diagnosis and determines the remedy. This could be an advantage if it left the doctor more time, in cases outside the present realm of science, to cultivate the relationship and exercise his art. It is tempting to think of the art of medicine as contracting, confined to the shrinking gaps where scientific knowledge is incomplete. But this would be quite wrong. Great skill and subtle judgment are required in applying science to an individual patient's illness. Science, by multiplying the choices, has immeasurably widened the scope of this art.

Scientific medicine has shifted the *context* of treatment towards the hospital and away from the home and the doctor's surgery. And scientific medicine is costly. Equipment becomes more complex and more expensive; hospitals year by year cost more to run. The newest developments—intensive care, automation, kidney machines and transplantation—make medicine costlier still. Scientific developments in medicine have not only presented society with a handsome and constantly increasing bill to pay and with a rumbustious pharmaceutical industry to control. They have also presented the elders of the profession and society the world over with a crop of new moral problems. These are discussed as they appear in turn in the narrative.

If drugs, science and technology are what most people would point to as the leading characteristic of medicine in recent decades, they share the credit with preventive medicine and with social and economic changes for the extraordinary fall in the mortality from infectious diseases. Deaths from these diseases in the age group 0–44 have fallen incredibly to one fortieth of the number forty years ago. Immunisation campaigns, against diphtheria, whooping cough, poliomyelitis and tuberculosis, responsible for part of this startling success, could not have been so successful unless medicine had used the opportunities for persuasion that modern media of communication have offered.

Developments in preventive medicine are described in Chapter 4 and these include two trends that are wholly of this century: the development of "screening", an attempt to uncover illness in its pre-symptomatic stage; and the steady growth of international institutions whose aim is to treat, control and prevent disease on a world-wide scale.

Although medicine with its scientific advances, its new drugs and its success in the prevention of infectious disease has bestowed so many benefits on mankind, it has saddled man, too, with some heavy burdens—the increasing cost of health, for example, and, as the fruit of its success, demands that effective cures, once discovered, shall be available to all. By far the most serious, however, is its contribution to three aspects of contemporary populations: sheer numbers; age-distribution; and quality. These subjects are discussed in Chapters 5 and 6.

The control of its population is perhaps the most urgent task that the world faces. The increase of between 2 and 3% a year continues and on current trends the present population is likely to double by the end of the century. Paradoxically, the more successful the efforts to improve international health by, for example, controlling malaria, and the greater the immediate aid in the form of food and drugs given by the richer to the poorer nations, the worse the situation becomes and the sharper the neo-Malthusian threat in some countries appears. Lord Caradon, a former Governor of Jamaica, has put the point succinctly ". . . if we endeavour to deal with the great world problems of poverty and hunger and ignorance and disease—and hatred and violence too—without at the same time dealing with the problem of population, we shall utterly fail."[1]

The remedies that we possess at present to check the growth in population—contraception, abortion and sterilisation—can be effective, as experience in Japan since the war has shown. Their application on a world scale is limited by difficulties in communication, by lack of education and by sheer lack of resources. They are hampered, too, by the opposition of most organised religions.

Some Western nations still have a need to control numbers. In others the demand for means to control fertility arises from new attitudes to child-rearing and from changing sexual mores. The demand is part and parcel of the self-assurance of mid-twentieth century man. He has convinced himself that an excess of political upheaval can be prevented by the democratic process and that post-Keynesian economics and a safety-net of social security will guarantee him a fair slice of a cake that grows slowly bigger—the so-called revolution of rising expectations. Medicine itself has removed the sudden threat of infectious diseases. Unwanted children are not only a menace to his new-found security, and a tyranny to his wife, but also, as he learns from the new psychology, will become the delinquents, the misfits and the neurotics of the next generation. Freudian psychology has probably convinced him, too, even if his own experience has not, that so powerful is the drive to expression of the sexual instinct that puritan methods of control, celibacy and continence are ineffectual except for the few.

Hence the demand for remedies—birth control not solely for medical reasons, nor solely for the married, abortion for purely social reasons, and sterilisation for the asking. There may well be sound social sense in these demands, but conflict could hardly be avoided with the conservative professions who guard society's conscience, the Church, the Law, and Medicine. The moral arguments need not specially concern us in this book. These demands, however, if granted will extend the concept of medicine and give new meanings to the words *doctor*, *patient* and *disease*. Doctors are necessarily involved in sterilisation and abortion and the newer and more efficient methods of contraception need their intervention too. They will find themselves doing operations which incur risk (and sometimes the taking of life) on well people, a role that many will shrink from. But since

[1] Reported in *The Lancet*, 29 April, 1967.

B

Jenner's time doctors have increasingly, in vaccination and inoculation, done just this to well people in the name of prevention.

Age-distribution has become the source of a number of problems since the steep decline in deaths from infectious diseases in the young and early middle-aged, and this has meant that more people nowadays survive to become elderly and aged. The age-distribution of the populations of wealthy countries has altered sharply. This "shift to the right", a greater probability that an ill person will also be an elderly person, with all the complications, social and psychiatric, that that can imply, has led to the development of the new specialty of geriatrics. At this extreme of life the borderline of medicine becomes shadowy. Concepts of *disease* and *patient*, who is regarded as sick and who as merely infirm, are in dispute, and at this extreme, too, a wealth of social factors join those more commonly regarded as medical as causes of disease.

The increase in number of the elderly in the population has had economic consequences as well. Coupled with modern medicine's capacity to save people from dying at the expense of increasing the number of the chronic sick, and with the effect of the spread of secondary and tertiary education, it has increased the ratio of the dependent to the productive in the total population.

There is also a fear that in tampering with the forces of natural selection medicine is dysgenic in its effect. It seems obvious that if medicine (and social policies) preserve the unfit from dying and enable them to reproduce, then, if there is a genetic component in these diseases, harmful genes will be preserved. But what may seem obvious is not necessarily true as examples in Chapter 6 show.

A strange assortment of influences has contributed to that other outstanding mid-century development in medicine—the growth of psychiatry. This phenomenon is described in Chapter 7. Some of these roots psychiatry has in common with the rest of medicine— effective drugs, for example, scientific methods of study and investigation, the stimulus of war, and the tardy realisation of the social causes of disease. Others are all its own. These certainly include psychological theories, notably those of Freud and Pavlov, and theories derived from the other behavioural sciences, particularly sociology, anthropology and animal ethology. It is paradoxical, however, that despite Freud's pervasive influence on society in general, on language, art, literature and on lay opinion about the springs of behaviour, clinical psychiatry, at least in England, owed as much and continues to owe a great deal to his contemporaries, the great nosologists: Emil Kraepelin at Heidelberg and Munich, who in 1883 named and described the disease groups dementia praecox and manic-depressive insanity; and Eugen Bleuler of Zürich, who proposed the concept of schizophrenia in 1911. American psychiatry, however, owes much more than psychiatry elsewhere to Freud's influence.

Psychiatry has grown not only in stature but also in scope, and in the process the concept of *disease* has expanded. Abnormal personalities hover on the brink of being regarded as sick, and diseases can now be defined in terms solely of disturbed behaviour. Medicine has already admitted many groups of offenders to its beds. Others are banging on the door and the principle of criminal responsibility is in danger of being shattered. At the same time psychiatry is heir to the declining church, which for the many has ceased to provide either faith, spiritual solace, or even social help. It is small wonder that, like medicine, psychiatry is itself in danger of fragmentation, its many branches employing concepts and a private technical language barely comprehensible to the others.

Fortunately, however, there are integrative forces in medicine, among them great ideas that shed a flood of light and make the links between the fragments, previously obscure, plain for all to see. In the past the germ theory of disease was one such; allergy was another. These remain, but "auto-intoxication" and "focal sepsis" have all but gone. Three twentieth century ideas of this type form the subject of Chapter 8: the concept of psychosomatic disease; the theory of stress diseases, which has links with the former; and the theory of auto-immunity and auto-immune disease.

It is a pity that "stress" has become a captive word, a prisoner of those who habitually use psychosomatic concepts. This has meant that it cannot be employed in a more natural sense without engendering confusion. It cannot be used, unless confusion is to be perpetuated, as a general term to describe the effects of extreme conditions on man's body and mind. Stresses of this sort, the limits of human endurance and the manner of human physical and psychological breakdown are described in Chapter 9. It could be objected that as applied physiology and experimental psychology these studies have no place in a book on medicine. They are, however, of great relevance, for there is hardly a frontier described—cold, compression, decompression, acceleration, deceleration, sensory deprivation—which does not border on some current medical preoccupation: accidental hypothermia in the elderly living alone; hyperbaric oxygen in the treatment of coal-gas poisoning and gas-

gangrene infection; deceleration research and road accidents;
sensory deprivation in night-driving and experimental psychosis.
Only weightlessness is really irrelevant, except for a handful of people,
but the subject, though unlikely to be experienced, is of sufficient
interest to merit a cursory inspection.

It is salutary but painful to reflect at this point on the stimulus that
war and preparation for war give to medical research. Much of the
work described in this chapter was paid for from military budgets;
even sensory deprivation experiments are related to psychological
warfare, brainwashing and defence against it. But medicine has
benefited time and again from the needs of war in this century.
Psychiatry has forged ahead in both world wars; orthopaedic surgery,
plastic surgery, and the treatment of burns gained immeasurably
from the Second World War; and would the large-scale manufacture
of penicillin have been achieved so quickly but for the war?

The last section of Chapter 9, dealing as it does with concentration camp existence, an existence characterised by extreme insecurity
and impoverishment, is of peculiar relevance. The diseases that were
common in these camps are those that Western societies have almost
extinguished—malnutrition and infections, including tuberculosis.
Those that were rare are precisely those that we are now plagued
with: asthma, peptic ulcers, hypertension, arterial disease, especially
coronary artery disease, and, incidentally, suicide and suicidal
attempts. There is a cosmic irony here; one imagines some malicious
gods laughing up their sleeves.

Some of our modern plagues, our diseases of affluence, are
described in Chapter 10. Their causes are largely unknown but are
almost certainly multiple, and therefore they can be expected to be
very difficult to eradicate. Many of them, addiction for example and
attempted suicide, again testify to how the concept of *disease* has
expanded in the last twenty years. Most have social and psychiatric
components. The diseases that they replace, infections and deficiencies, had almost single causes. But there is hope. Pulmonary tuberculosis, though the presence of the tubercle bacillus was essential,
was long regarded as essentially a complex disease with genetic,
psychosomatic, and social causes. Deaths from this disease in England
have nevertheless fallen from 32,000 to 1,844 in forty years.

These vast changes in medicine, changes in the concept of disease
and changes in disease frequency, changes in the role of the doctor,
changes in the patient—in the sort of person he is, in the sort of
problem he brings—and changes in the relationship, might have been
expected to call for a most radical revision of the doctor's training.

By and large medical education has kept abreast of technical development, of pharmaceutical prowess, and to some extent of developments in psychiatry. But in other respects—and this is the subject of Chapter 11—the student is being trained, and not only in England, for the practice of a generation ago. Unless he corrects his training by his own untutored exertions he is likely to be ignorant of developments in general practice, preventive medicine, geriatrics, and community medicine, fit only to follow in the footsteps of his clinical chiefs.

The final chapter—Chapter 12—deals with the *context* in which medicine is practised, in Britain and in other countries, with the strains that the continually rising cost of health has imposed and with the increasing part that health insurance and central government finance have consequently had to play.

This book, to sum up, aims at something more than a study of the changes that have taken place in the fundamental terms of the medical equation, though these are startling enough. It tries to relate these changes to the changed setting, to the characteristics of a world on which Marx and Keynes, Freud and Fleming, have left their imprint; a world where, at least in some countries, egalitarian ideas are in the ascendant, economic advance is taken for granted, and people have rising expectations and expect, moreover, the state to cushion them in adversity from want and disease a world in which— to overstate for the moment in order to make the point—morality is permissive, anything goes, philosophy is materialist, determinist or hedonist and God is only the subject of an argument. All's well except for the shadow of a mushroom cloud. But to return: the book also attempts to draw attention to modern medicine's consequences, to the economic, social, and again and again the ethical problems that medicine has created and which society will need to solve.

CHAPTER TWO

Science, Technology and Experimental Medicine

The Invasion by Science

The explosion of scientific knowledge since the Second World War is said to be fiercer than the population explosion. The rate of acceleration is still increasing. Certainly, science dominates medicine now to an extent undreamed of even fifty years ago and medical progress in this century far outstrips that of all previous centuries put together. All the branches of medicine have been transformed out of all recognition. The triumph of the starched white coat has been complete and the trappings of an older medicine, the frock coat, the stock, and the wing collar, have gone into the dustbin.

This triumph is symptomatic of a deeper change in society. Authority-figures have lost esteem in our permissive society and the frock-coated doctor, whose authority was derived in part from a quasi-priestly training, has vanished with them. Insofar as anyone is revered today it is the expert, particularly the scientist—agnostic, amoral—who, if he makes any moral judgments (as a scientist) at all, equates good with biological adaptation and bad with maladaptation. Disease, then, is failure to adapt. The scientifically trained doctor is in a quandary when faced with a patient. He sees him both as a failing organism and as a sick and suffering person. It is perhaps surprising that more of the humanity of doctors has not accompanied the frock coat into the dustbin.

White-coat medicine for all its heady achievements—and it has been overwhelmingly beneficial—has had its drawbacks. It has filched the limelight; and white-coat medicine means hospital medicine. The other branches are in the shadow—general practice, preventive medicine, community medicine. They have no réclame in the public's estimation and—as important for medicine's future—in the estimation of future doctors. Science's own child, experimental medicine, is no little innocent. In its passion for experiment it has presented society with troublesome ethical problems—and a sizeable bill to pay.

To do justice to science's impact on medicine, to chart how each and every branch has been affected, would be a Herculean task. To select examples risks the criticism that more important ones have been left out. It is plain, however, that the benefits are manifold and manifest and that without them many of us would be dead. One takes for granted that the flow will continue: this week a new application of lasers in surgery; next week a triumph for hyperbaric oxygen, a new method of studying some disease by radio-isotopes, a new plastic for heart valve replacement, a fresh syndrome recognised by chromosome analysis. There is no sign, as there is in the discovery of new drugs, of the source drying up.

Even the shortest list must include:

Physiological research in the field of anaesthesia. This underlies all modern surgery and has made open heart surgery possible.

The biochemical analysis of every body fluid and the light this has thrown on a hundred diseases ranging from diabetes to the inborn errors of metabolism.

The development of machines—the electrocardiograph, the electroencephalograph and the electromyograph—to trace the electrical activities of body tissues for use in clinical diagnosis.

The invention of metals and polymers suitable for use in orthopaedic and arterial surgery.

The advances of haemotology and immunology: the former of cardinal importance in the investigation of a host of diseases not only of the blood; the latter in, for example, Rh iso-immunisation and transplant surgery.

Discoveries in physics leading to the construction of even more sophisticated machines for the treatment of cancer.

The use of statistics as a research weapon.

Medicine, moreover, has not been content just to use the products of science; it also directly employs a growing army of scientists and technicians on its own account: biochemists, physicists, electrocardiograph and electroencephalograph technicians and those trained to handle radio-isotopes.

A few aspects of scientific medicine need closer examination because they signify fundamental changes in the practice of medicine or because they reflect new problems for society—economic, political, ethical—problems peculiar to this century.

The Ascendancy of the Laboratory

Few patients today are admitted to hospital without undergoing a series, often quite a long series, of investigations. Year by year informative new tests are added. The eyes, ears and fingertips of the physician, aided by a few simple instruments, which had to suffice in former centuries, now have this powerful supplement.

Some laboratories report that the work load seems to double every five years and there is no sign of any levelling-off. The reasons are not obscure and may be summarised quite easily: more patients from a growing population attend; more investigations are possible; new treatments have been invented which require laboratory control— for example, during anticoagulant therapy in coronary artery disease and the use of cytotoxic drugs in cancer; new demands have arisen for screening of populations—for example, cervical smears of all women over thirty, routine examinations of sputum for cancer cells in smokers, examination of the urine of those employed in trades where there is a risk of bladder cancer. It is the growth of techniques for screening segments of the population that makes clinical pathologists doubtful if their work will ever stop expanding.

The insistent demand for an increase in technical staff to cope with this extra work is, with the ever-increasing drug bill, contributing handsomely to the rising cost of medicine. To a very limited extent a few investigations are being handed back to the clinician; with impregnated paper he can now test babies for phenylketonuria (though this test has been criticised) and test his patients, particularly his diabetic patients, for abnormal levels of sugar in the blood.

One reason for the discontent of the general practitioner is the limited access that he has to laboratories. His liberty to practise the kind of medicine that he has been taught is thereby curtailed; he is fighting disease with one hand behind his back.

Automation and Computers

The great hope of the future in chemical pathology lies in automation. Already machines exist that can count the number of cells in a sample of blood. Others can automatically carry out the laborious steps of staining blood films, can estimate the amount of haemoglobin, can measure simultaneously the levels of four electrolytes in the blood, and can even determine blood groups.

Development of automation in laboratory work requires a lot of capital—a multichannel blood counting and blood grouping machine costs £5,000–£6,000. Even more versatile machines are on the market. One multichannel machine can measure twelve different blood constituents in ten minutes and process 300 blood samples in an hour. The cost, £15,000–£30,000, might be an economy if, as reported,[1] this machine saves the work of sixty technicians. Machines such as these, already in wide use in the United States, save dreary routine work and they are more accurate than technicians. They ensure that routine blood and chemical investigation can be carried out on every patient for little extra cost and, if employed on out-patients, might save many patients from having to be admitted to hospital at all—potentially a very great economy.

Even more time could probably be saved by the application of machines to the recording of results, the issuing of reports and storage of data. Computer firms are well aware[2] of the potentiality of this new field.

Much more far-reaching is the Ministry of Health's plan[3] to install computers in two London hospitals. With this, medicine in Britain will enter a new era.

Until now, as an enthusiast for medical automation has pointed out,[4] one man's knowledge, experience and judgment, his "intuition" and his clinical acumen were the most that could be brought to bear on a clinical problem. This, in fact, is the essence of consultant practice. The storage capacity of modern computers enables the knowledge and experience of innumerable other clinicians to be brought in. The computer does demand, however, that information should be provided in a usable form. If, as many people think, we are on the threshold of a revolution in the application of computers and automation to medical problems there will have first to be big changes in recording details of patients' medical histories and of clinical examination. Check-lists may oust the narrative form. No amount of machinery can, however, compensate for inaccurate and incomplete clinical observation.

More basically the permeation of medicine by automation and computers will compel a change in habits of thought and in medical education. "The brightest academics in medicine will soon be more interested in mathematics and cybernetics than in today's fashionable molecular biology . . ."[5]

[1] *Guardian*, 15 February, 1968.
[2] *Report of a Conference on Data-processing and Computer Techniques in Clinical Biochemistry. Lancet* (1965), **i,** 1111.
[3] *The Times*, 15 February, 1968.
[4] Payne, L. C. *An Introduction to Medical Automation*. (Pitman Medical Publishing. London, 1966).
[5] Burnet, F. M. (1964), *Brit. Med. J.*, **ii,** 1091.

Intensive Care

Although units known as intensive care or intensive therapy units have been in use for several years in Britain and elsewhere, there is as yet little unanimity about their definition, or what sort of condition should be cared for and treated in them, or, indeed, on who should be in charge of them. They developed from the respiratory units used in treating patients with paralysis of breathing in the poliomyelitis epidemics of the early 1950s, and some authors define the suitable patient as one who requires "the mechanical support of a vital function until the disease process is corrected or ameliorated"[1] —the heart, the lungs, the kidneys. People likely to be admitted include those recovering from major heart and chest surgery, patients with chest injuries from road accidents, those with acute renal failure, severe coronary thrombosis, prolonged coma from poisoning, severe burns, severe tetanus and severe blood loss. Everyone agrees that an intensive therapy unit worth the name needs much space for few beds, ample highly trained nursing staff, its own laboratory, sophisticated equipment, and probably extensive and expensive monitoring facilities to watch vital functions.

For others the phrase implies only a place for looking after patients who need medical and nursing attention beyond the resources of ordinary wards, or, in surgery, a rather more elaborate recovery ward than usual. Some, perhaps most, see a need for the great majority of those admitted to stay for only a short period—two to four days—but in one unit the average stay is almost three weeks. As for who should be in charge the majority seem to favour an anaesthetist, whereas others say either that the unit should be run by a clinical physiologist or that each patient in the unit should remain in the care of his own physician or surgeon.

There seems to be agreement that these units save lives,[2] [3] though one author at least does not agree and adds, "One is tempted to say that treatment is often more intense than careful."[4] There is no evidence, however, that a unit saves nursing elsewhere in the hospital. Both the capital cost and the running costs are high.

Even more specialised intensive treatment units are in the wind. "A coronary care unit is an important factor in reducing mortality from myocardial infarction. Such units should be established in all large hospitals dealing with acute cases",[5] advice that was anticipated

[1] Robinson, J S. (1966), *Proc. Roy. Soc. Med.*, **59**, 1293.
[2] Ibid.
[3] Lees, W. (1965), *Lancet*, **ii**, 285.
[4] Dornhorst, A. C. (1966), *Proc. Roy. Soc. Med.*, **59**, 1293.
[5] Goble, A. J., Sloman, G. and Robinson, J. S. (1966), *Brit. Med. J.*, **i**, 1005.

and is being widely followed in progressive hospitals in advanced countries. Upwards of three-fifths of the deaths from coronary thrombosis occur in the first week after the attack. Many of these cannot be prevented even with the most advanced techniques. But others can, and so can many deaths occurring later if monitoring is persistent and if all the necessary machinery for resuscitation and skilled nurses and doctors are immediately available.

Coronary attacks are not only increasing in frequency. They are spreading to younger age groups (see Chapter 10). The disease is particularly common in men of social classes I and II. If the critical research into the effectiveness of coronary care units pleaded for[1] really does show that they save life the demand for their widespread establishment will become both medically and politically irresistible. The cost will be high in terms of equipment and of the numbers of trained nurses required. At a time when there are already too few doctors in Britain for all the tasks to be done, and when of all the middle and junior posts in hospital 44% are filled by graduates from overseas[2] the extra load these units would cause might be insupportable. Yet, unless they are properly staffed they will fail and the principle of intensive therapy will be discredited. If we will the end we must somehow will the means.

Haemodialysis and Kidney Transplantation

Articles by the hundred in the world medical press and by the score in the lay press testify to the enormous interest that these two new methods of treating chronic renal failure have aroused. Only very recently has interest shifted, as techniques have improved, from the medical, surgical, technical and immunological aspects to the economic and ethical.

Haemodialysis as a form of treatment developed out of Kolff's experiments with the artificial kidney in Holland in the late 1940s. Its use in acute renal failure and in removing poisons rapidly from the circulation, for example in barbiturate coma, is uncontroversial. Chronic dialysis, pioneered by Scribner in Seattle in 1960, aims at keeping alive and in good working health sufferers from chronic kidney failure in whom dietary treatment has failed and who otherwise would very soon die from uraemia. Figures for Europe showed that of 1,163 patients accepted for dialysis by May, 1967, 376 had died. The remainder were still on dialysis or had been transplanted.

[1] Shillingford, J. P. (1966), *Brit. Med. J.*, **1,** 1047.
[2] *Lancet*, 15 July, 1967, p. 159 refers to the situation in September, 1966.

Established centres are even more successful. In June 1966, some of Scribner's patients were still alive in their seventh year, and elsewhere people have lived for more than five years with twice-a-week dialysis. The Seattle centre has treated 23 patients for 40 patient-years with three deaths;[1] two London centres report 35 patients treated for 43 patient years with only one death;[2] and similar results come from other experienced centres.

Yet formidable difficulties and dangers remain—side-effects of the treatment, epidemics of hepatitis such as have happened in Seattle and Manchester with deaths among patients and staff, and problems with clotting in the permanently indwelling arteriovenous shunt. Life on dialysis is no picnic. Home dialysis and disposable artificial kidneys are newer developments, each with its own special difficulties.

Renal transplantation, too, where the main problem has always been to prevent the natural immune defences of the body from destroying the graft,[3] has been advancing. The first successful kidney transplant (between identical twins) was done by Murray, Merrill and Harrison as recently as 1954.[4] Pooled world results up to March, 1965 showed that of 392 recipients of transplants only 37% were living a year later.[5] But here again, in transplantation centres with the best results 70–80% of grafts from near relatives and 50% of those from dead bodies were surviving at the end of a year.[6] No doubt improvements in tissue-typing will enable a more compatible graft to be chosen and there may well be further progress in immunosuppression—by drugs and the newer anti-lymphocytic serum—so that not only will the life of the graft and the patient be prolonged, but the risk of lethal infection (always present with these drugs) will be diminished as well.

Nevertheless, 7,000 or so people die of renal failure each year in England and Wales and 3,000 of them die between the ages of five and fifty-five. For a variety of reasons many of these would be unsuitable candidates for intermittent dialysis, and estimates of the numbers of suitable new cases arising each year range from 1,500 to 2,500. In America a similar estimate is 10,000.[7]

[1] Pendras, J. P. and Erickson, R. V. (1966), *Ann. Intern. Med.*, **64**, 293.
[2] de Wardener, H. E. in *Ethics in Medical Progress*. Ciba Foundation Symposium. ed. G. E. W. Wolstenholme and M. O'Connor. (Churchill. London, 1966).
[3] This is hardly a problem in corneal grafting for the cornea has no blood supply; for the same reason the eye to be used for grafting does not, unlike the kidney, have to be removed from the body within a few minutes of death.
[4] Murray, J. E., Merrill, J. P. and Harrison, J. H. (1955), *Surg. Forum.*, **6**, 432.
[5] By January 1968 1,741 transplants had been done with more survivals among the later cases.
[6] Calne, R. Y. (1966), *Proc. Roy. Soc. Med.*, **59**, 670.
[7] Murray, J. E. in *Ethics in Medical Progress*.

The capital cost of the equipment needed for one bed for dialysis in hospital is about £1,500 a year—i.e. about £500 per patient on twice-a-week maintenance dialysis. If the maintenance costs are added the total cost per patient could well amount to £1,800 per year. On the pessimistic assumption that only 50% of patients taken on for treatment are still having it at the end of five years the annual maintenance costs might, for 11,000 patients, amount to £16 million and in addition capital costs of £7 million would have been incurred.[1] Optimistic assumptions about survival lead to much higher estimates.

The present plan in Britain is to open 20 main dialysis centres capable of maintaining approximately 600 patients on dialysis twice a week. These will clearly satisfy only a small proportion of the accumulating need. They will fill up rapidly as they are opened. New and suitable patients will continue to find, as now, that there is no place for them. But, even if money and machines were suddenly conjured up to the limit, the shortage of skilled staff would cripple the programme.

It is very unfortunate that these two forms of treatment for the same condition should have developed to some extent in competition; it is tragic that someone who has graduated from his machine to a transplant that then fails should find the dialysis machine occupied by someone else when he again needs it. But surely this is inevitable with the present shortage. Clearly the treatments are complementary. The ultimate aim should be a properly functioning graft. The role of dialysis is to improve the patient's condition before operation and to make him fit for it. If the operation is a failure he will need his machine again till a more successful graft is forthcoming. But, again, the number of transplantation operations in Britain each year — increased as it may be by the opening of new renal transplantation centres to perhaps 600 operations—will only supply a fraction of the need. This fraction would be higher if the "take" rate of cadaver kidneys, the least troublesome source but at present the least successful, could be raised, and if the life of grafts could be prolonged.

More than most areas of medicine, more perhaps than psychiatry and geriatrics and population problems, these two topics are ringed with political, economic, social and ethical mines and booby traps. Is a truly adequate haemodialysis programme within the present resources of the health service worth three new district hospitals? If it is added to the current programme—not to mention the cost of 150 intensive care units—do we forgo x aeroplanes in the defence pro-

[1] de Wardener, H. E., op. cit.

gramme or *y* new schools? If shortages persist, who is to choose the
survivors and to condemn the rest to death on the grounds of being
"unsuitable"? Or is there to be some kind of board so that, in matters
of life and death, doctors can shed their responsibility for choosing
into laymen's laps—a craven retreat surely? Granted that grafts
from relations have the best chance of success, who is to ensure
that potential donors are not under extreme pressure from conscience
and from other relatives? In fact, is a living donor an ethically
acceptable proposition? Should an operation with both immediate
and long term risks be done on well people? "Some biologically
suitable donors can and do make it clear that they don't want to
offer a kidney. They don't necessarily have to say so in so many
words—they make it quite apparent and at the slightest evidence of
this we just say they are unacceptable for technical reasons . . . We
never accept a 'yes' at our first discussion."[1] If cadavers are a less
unsatisfactory source how to ensure that their kidney can be obtained
within a few minutes of death so that it has not deteriorated to the
point of being useless? Are preparations to be made such as the
taking of blood for tissue typing as soon as it is known that a suitable
person is going to die—the transplantation team hovering like
vultures? When, nowadays, are some people in fact dead? The
moment has become more difficult to define. But, certainly, some
new Act will be necessary, or some clarification of the Human Tissue
Act of 1961, which will allow hospital authorities to remove organs
from a body immediately after death unless the next of kin object
immediately or unless the donor, in life, forbade it.

Somewhat similar choices have been forced on the medical profession before—with penicillin in the war, with streptomycin in
tuberculosis and with cortisone in its early days, but in these cases
(with the exception of tuberculous meningitis and miliary tuberculosis) the choice was never quite so starkly between life and death;
there were other established and quite effective remedies. One
wonders whether, if a tithe of the money that it is proposed to devote
to the treatment of chronic kidney failure were invested in trying to
find out its causes, all these dilemmas and heartaches might not vanish.

Heart Transplantation

This even newer achievement of scientific medicine has shown that
compared with kidney transplantation there are additional difficulties. The technical achievement is greater; the problem of immunity

[1] Woodruff, M. F. A. (1966), *Ethics in Medical Progress.*

and graft-rejection is the same; the recipient is likely to be in less good shape because there is no device akin to the artificial kidney to improve his physical condition before operation. Equally, because there is no dialysis machine to retire to if the operation fails, the heart operation has a much more dramatic quality as a gambler's last throw, a quality that the heart, because of its symbolic meaning, already possesses. Perhaps this goes some way towards accounting for the intense public interest in the early heart transplantation operations.

It is true that the ethical problem of the healthy donor does not arise, but the same speed is necessary and it has become plainer than ever that the potential donor must be cared for by a set of doctors entirely independent of the transplantation team. Indeed, in many countries this division is incorporated in professional policy.

A start has been made with transplantation of human liver and lungs. Perhaps the complexities of immunology will be unravelled so that grafts from animals can take. If so, many current ethical perplexities will melt away. At present, if only because central nervous system tissue does not regenerate, brain-grafting appears to be quite impossible. If it were possible, society's present moral quandaries about transplantation would in comparison pale into insignificance. As things are, man appears to be faced with the prospect of being given a fresh lease of life from a new heart or liver while his brain continues to run down. Is this what he wants and what he is likely to will?

Experimental Medicine

The previous section has shown that medicine has made good use of the fruits of scientific knowledge, and in transplant surgery the most exotic fruit. It does not follow that the methods of science have been nearly so pervasive. Medicine is not much nearer to being only applied science than it was at the beginning of the century and doctors still uncomfortably bestride the two cultures.

The scientific method, insofar as it consists of observation, the classification of phenomena, measurement, hypothesis and inductive reasoning, has been used in medicine for centuries. Insofar as it involves experiment, medicine applies it with great caution, and the philosophical foundation of the scientist, the conviction that nothing is finally proved and that one fresh fact can always upset a firmly established hypothesis, is alien to the doctor as healer. The physician, too, uses methods other than the scientific for gathering information and evaluating it. He sets great store by the history of the patient and of his illness, and in judging how reliable the various sources of information are he makes value-judgments in the manner more of a historian than of a scientist. As a healer he is aware of the importance of many truths which science as yet cannot begin to fathom: that in dealing with human beings phenomena may alter solely because they are being observed and measured; that the relationship between a patient and his doctor, which is quite unmeasurable, may be crucial in deciding the outcome of an illness; that hopes and fears and confidence can be of immense importance; and that the effect of a remedy may be determined by who gives it or by what the patient believes it to contain rather than by its inherent properties. In his Harveian Oration of 1964, Professor Sir George Pickering[1] remarked:

"In fact, in my youth I often noted a certain hostility between physicians and scientists—particularly those whose enquiries had led them to, or near to, a study of disease in man. I have often wondered whether there is an antipathy between the roles of physician and scientist; if so, what is the nature of this antipathy; and whether it is inherent in these two occupations."

The fact is that most doctors play both roles. All have a basic training in the methods of science and many retain the scientific attitude to their work. They continue to observe, to record, to classify and to measure—all the more now since science is continually providing new methods of observation and of measurement and new techniques of recording. The conflict comes at a later stage in trying to treat the patient's illness. Here many doctors find it unacceptable to perform experiments even if the impact of that word is softened by calling them "a controlled trial". No doubt sometimes he can in Sir George's words "deliberately alter one factor at a time to see if, and in what way, this alteration affects the result", but often he cannot, particularly if the factor is a remedy which he rightly or wrongly believes will help the patient and the "alteration" means that the patient is given nothing.

The rift indeed goes deeper than this. The scepticism of the scientist is alarming to any patient who fears that he may have some serious illness, and for this reason not many first-rate scientists have made good doctors. On the other hand, the credulity and faith of the doctor communicate themselves to the patient and are in themselves therapeutic. He gets better though he has no reason known to science to do so. The discarded remedies of past decades did undoubtedly help large numbers of patients although we know that there was no virtue in the remedies themselves.

[1] Pickering, Sir George. (1964), "Physician and Scientist." *Brit. Med. J.*, **ii,** 1615.

There is a dilemma here which the march of science has made more acute. It is a moral one and concerns the justification of means by ends. Medicine is in a post-Linnaean era, and most of the observation, description and classification has been done, although the occasional brilliant observation is still made and new syndromes caused by biochemical and chromosomal abnormalities are still being recognised. Major advances in medicine can, in the main, be made only in the scientific fields of measurement and experimental therapeutics. Animal experiments do not get very far and the results can be dangerously misleading. The unpleasant fact is that medicine can advance only by means of experiments on human beings—call these experiments what you will—and that if these are not made it will stagnate. But it will languish in a state of dangerous pseudo-empiricism. Potent half-tried remedies will continue to emerge and may be used for years before anyone is sure that they are useful or before they are discarded.

The history of deep insulin treatment for schizophrenia is a cautionary example. It was introduced in Vienna in 1933 and was difficult to apply and very expensive in terms of medical and nursing care. Its use, on the basis of many favourable reports, spread to all the advanced countries of the world, but few psychiatrists were wholly convinced that these favourable reports were entirely reliable. It was not until 1957 that a report of a trial using barbiturate-induced coma in controls was published[1] and showed that the insulin-treated patients gained no advantage. It is probable that the publication of the results of this trial would on its own have convinced most psychiatrists that the therapy should be given up, although some enthusiasts, no doubt, would have clung to it. The success of an alternative method of treatment—the use of the phenothiazine group of drugs—resolved all doubts and in Britain insulin coma treatment is now seldom used.

The alternative to treatment based on inadequate knowledge is the properly designed clinical trial, designed expressly to give a once and for all answer to the question of whether a newly introduced remedy is effective or not. This is as characteristic of our time as were the classic descriptions of diseases of an earlier epoch, and it is parallele in the non-medical sphere by the quasi-scientific tests of consumer products. Not every doctor agrees with the principle and only a minority of doctors take part or encourage their patients—fully apprised and willing though they may be—to participate; but everyone makes use of the answers, and these rapidly acquire authority and

[1] Ackner, B., Harris, A. and Oldham, A J. (1957), *Lancet*, **i,** 607.

C

enter the archives of that organised body of knowledge which is the foundation of the practice of medicine. If doctors applaud the ends and use them must they necessarily endorse the means?

In therapeutics the deliberate design of a human experiment and the use of statistical methods are by no means new. In 1747 Lind was experimenting with six different forms of treatment for scurvy on twelve patients. Only the two people who had two oranges and a lemon each day got better. What is new in the last thirty years is a spreading awareness that in trials of new treatments only properly designed experiments will yield useful and repeatable results. It is not so much that these trials have become the fashion as that people have become aware that any other kind of trial is so full of pitfalls that no reliable information can be gleaned from it. There are exceptions of course. A few diseases have had a 100% mortality. Any remedy which saved the patient, such as streptomycin given to someone with tuberculous meningitis, must have been effective; no planning or statistical manipulation was needed to show this—only one patient's survival.

But most illnesses are much less certain in their outcome, and to show for sure that one remedy has an advantage over another or over no treatment at all is often a matter of great difficulty.

First, the phenomena must be truly comparable, the patients in the two groups firmly diagnosed so far as is possible and the illnesses homogeneous. The patients must be equally severely affected and evenly matched in other respects that might affect the outcome— age, sex, racial origin, social class, etc. They must be having similar nursing care, in similar environments, the same diet and the same kinds of accessory treatment. The aim is to control all the other variables except the specific therapy in question.

Secondly, it is crucial to try to eliminate the possibility that the apparent advantage of one form of treatment over another kind or over no treatment at all could be quite easily due to chance. In theory even an exceedingly unlikely event could possibly be due to chance; therefore the problem is to define in mathematical terms the probability of any difference being a chance difference. This probability depends both on how striking is the contrast in outcome and on how many patients are involved, and therefore, in many well-designed trials, a pilot study is carried out first. This may indicate the likely degree of difference in outcome so that the number of patients needed for an arbitrarily defined level of "significance" to emerge can be tentatively estimated. A fairly new and sophisticated statistical technique—sequential analysis—eliminates this step. In this method of comparison between two therapies patients are added to the trial step by step till a generally accepted "significant" difference between treatments eventually does or does not emerge. This method is particularly suited to a clinical experimenter dealing with a fairly uncommon illness. Patients can be added to his trial as they crop up over a period of two or three years. The alternative method of dealing with uncommon illnesses is the large-scale trial involving many different hospitals so that a sufficient number of patients is in the trial. This solution is open to the objection that the rule of *ceteris paribus* is breached. Nursing care, diet and surroundings are bound to be different—but perhaps not so different as to affect the result.

These two hazards of non-comparability and chance are hazards of animal experiments as well. The remaining two are peculiarly human. The first is in the psychology of the experimenter. He is no more immune to hopes, fears and prejudice than the rest of us, particularly when he is treating sick people with unpleasant illnesses. His bias can consciously or unconsciously affect the results of a trial. He may allocate the more sick patients to the group having the treatment that he thinks is more effective, or he may overestimate or underestimate the effects of treatment. For this reason in strictly controlled trials the patients are randomly allocated to the various treatment groups or to the no-treatment group (if the conscience of the experimenter allows him to have one) and the experimenter should have no knowledge, at the time he is assessing progress, of what treatment any particular patient is having. Usually it is the hospital pharmacist who has the code locked away in his dispensary. The same rule, of course, applies to nurses if they are asked to assess progress. This is one blinker of the double-blind trial.

The other is that the patient must not know what treatment, if any, he is having. This is even more important, and in all experimental trials of this type the patients, of whatever treatment group even if they are having none, are given identical-looking tablets or capsules. The tablet or capsule containing no active ingredients is called a placebo and is a potent weapon in modern experimental medicine.

Placebos, Double-blind Trials and Ethics

The dictionary[1] definition of a placebo as "a medicine given more to please than to benefit the patient—1811" sounds old-fashioned today, for the word is seldom used nowadays outside the context of

[1] *The Shorter Oxford English Dictionary.* (Clarendon Press, Oxford, 1944. 3rd ed.).

the therapeutic trial. We are now more interested in the benefits, for it has been quite conclusively shown that the placebo can be powerfully therapeutic. In a piece of research published in 1933[1] on drugs used in angina pectoris 37·5% of the patients showed great or moderate improvement in their symptoms on a placebo, a higher proportion than on any of sixteen drugs then in use for treating this condition. Since then many studies have shown again and again that symptoms of quite serious diseases can be greatly relieved in 30–40% of cases by placebos, and oddly enough that they are more effective in relieving severe symptoms than mild ones.[2]

People who respond to placebos are equally of either sex and of average intelligence, but they tend to be older, more anxious and more preoccupied by their own bodily processes than those who do not react. Placebos can produce observable side-effects like rashes or a change in gastric secretion, but in general they are more effective in relieving subjective symptoms, and the high successes of placebos have mostly been recorded in the treatment of such symptoms as seasickness, anxiety, cough, post-operative wound pain, headache, and in the common cold.

How they work is a mystery and one is little farther forward in invoking "suggestion" or, more psychoanalytically, "the placebo acts by symbolically supplying for the adult that which during infancy was supplied by the mother", that is milk.[3] What is quite clear is that it is right to suspect any report of research into a new drug which shows that it cannot relieve more than 40% of patients.

This picture of the ideal controlled double-blind trial is frequently impossible to achieve in practice. Unnecessary operations or even painful investigations cannot be done on healthy controls; many drugs have side-effects that make it obvious to both patient and doctor that a placebo is not being used; in serious illnesses a placebo-group or a no-treatment group would be unthinkable. Nevertheless thought, design and ingenuity can often evade these difficulties and produce "hard" information.

The wide use of statistical methods in British medicine dates from Sir Austin Bradford Hill's articles in the *Lancet* in 1936, later published as a book.[4] The fruits include a series of designed large-scale trials organised by the Medical Research Council, starting with the convincing demonstration of the value of streptomycin in pulmonary

[1] Evans, W. and Hoyle, C. (1933), *Quart. J. Med.*, **26**, 311.
[2] Lassagna, L., Mosteller, F., Felsinger, J. M. and Beecher, H. J. (1954), *Amer. J. Med* **16**, 770.
[3] Forrer, G. R. (1964), *Dis. Nerv. System*, **25**, 655.
[4] Bradford Hill, A. *Principles of Medical Statistics*. (Lancet. London, 1937).

tuberculosis published in 1948,[1] and a swelling volume of other statistically respectable research. Today medical research has been thoroughly permeated by statistical design, and potential authors risk finding the editors of journals adamantly refusing to accept work for publication in which these principles have been ignored. Much of the work published in medical journals is not suited to the use of a statistical approach—descriptions of new syndromes and diseases, new techniques and kinds of treatment, fresh forms of investigation, and historical material. But where it is appropriate it is usually required.

Nevertheless the invasion of medicine by statistical methods has not been unopposed. In part this has reflected a widespread scepticism of the worth of expertise expressed in the "you can prove anything by statistics" phrase; in part it derives from a misunderstanding of what these methods can and cannot do. They can yield evidence of association but not of cause, and the gap leaves ample room for argument. The history of the controversy over smoking and cancer of the lung, which raged for years after the evidence of an association between them was first published,[2] is probably the best example of this, and a splendid lesson, too, in the enmity between scientific knowledge and strong emotion.

Other criticisms have been made: of the use of sophisticated statistical techniques that only a few readers of the published results can understand; of the air of spurious accuracy that is given when these techniques are applied to inadequate data; and of the devaluation that excellent clinical observation has suffered. The double-blind control trial has come in for particular criticism.[3] Many of the points concerning fixed doses, rigid time-schedules, the sensitiveness of the grading of response, and the consequences of side-effects on the blindness and double-blindness of the trial apply to drugs used in many different diseases; but they are at their most telling in trials of drugs used in psychiatry. The antidepressant and, even more, the tranquillising antipsychotic drugs have a huge range of effective dose—some patients respond to small and others only to vast doses; they can often work perfectly satisfactorily after a long delay; they produce side-effects when used in adequate dosage; and the response to them is difficult to grade. The conditions of the trial, too, the extra observation and attention, the altered attitude of the nursing

[1] Report of the Streptomycin in Tuberculosis Trials Committee (1948). *Brit. Med. J.*, **ii,** 769.
[2] Doll, W. R. and Hill, A. Bradford. (1950), *Brit. Med. J.*, **ii,** 739.
[3] Cromie, B. W. (1963), *Lancet*, **ii,** 994.

staff can influence both the trial and the control patients and dilute any differences between them.

One last criticism can legitimately be made of some controlled trials. The patient may be told or unwittingly led to believe that he is having a form of treatment when, in fact, the doctor in charge knows that half the people in the trial are having a placebo. To quote from a recent report as a typical example:

"Each patient was told at the start of the trial that there was no treatment that could be guaranteed to keep him well, but that we were trying various remedies for this purpose . . . patients were given a prescription as follows:—[name of drug] maintenance trial 0·5 G. q.d.s. The patients were then randomly allocated by the pharmacist into either the active-treatment group or the placebo group, so that neither the patient nor the doctor knew the nature of the treatment given."

Lies have sometimes to be told to patients with serious diseases like cancer, but it seems that half the people in this trial had deliberately been led to believe that they were having a form of treatment when, in fact, they were not. Nevertheless the trial showed that the drug was unequivocally superior to a placebo.

A more debatable point arises from an M.R.C. clinical trial of the treatment of depressive illness.[1] In this the patients knew that they might be receiving one of three types of treatment or no treatment for a month and they were told the truth. On the other hand their doctors considered them all to be sufficiently ill to be given E.C.T. (Electric Convulsive Therapy) if they fell randomly into the group allocated to this treatment and yet could contemplate their having a placebo for a month if they fell into that group. Depression is an exceedingly unpleasant frame of mind, with suicide an ever-present risk, and all these patients were considered ill enough to be in hospital. It is true that the doctors had the right to change the treatment if they felt the clinical necessity to do so. "To comfort always"? Fortunately nobody died, at least in the four weeks when placebos were being used, but had one of the group having a placebo committed suicide there would have been some shamed faces and a bereaved family. The results of the trial were clear, unequivocal and valuable, but the pursuit of science leads doctors up some questionable alleyways.

It is easy enough to disapprove of the human experiments made in concentration camps in Germany, which, in any case, seem to

[1] *Brit. Med. J.* (1965), **i,** 881.

have been curiously unfruitful. Our moral dilemma is much more subtle. The end, the definitive delimitation of the field of usefulness of a new drug and of its dangers, is praiseworthy, and useful drugs can then with speed and confidence be applied to the relief of patients far and wide. The means is the problem, and only if the means is known in all its intricacy can the public decide whether it is justifiable.

We need to be vigilant. Human sacrifice in a subtle and muted form has reappeared, this time on the altar of science. "Volunteers" are easy to obtain: patients who trust their doctors and want to please them consent; students freshly attired in the mantle of science consent; in some countries prisoners with a promise of early release consent. Worse still the subnormal or the chronic mentally ill have no opportunity to dissent. It is true that in Britain such groups are not as a rule employed in these experiments until the experimenter himself and perhaps some of his colleagues, who are the people most likely to be fully aware of all the risks, have themselves tried the drug.

Those who are unaware of the excesses of experimental medicine and of the hair-raising things that are sometimes done to people in its name—patients, controls, children, students, prisoners, the mentally ill and subnormal—would be enlightened by a recently published book.[1]

Since, as citizens and potential patients, we are more than willing to accept the advances of therapeutics with open arms we have also to accept the responsibility for the means by which such advances are made. But, again, we need to be vigilant and to know what is being done on our behalf. The scientist in the doctor needs watching.

[1] Pappworth, M. H. *Human Guinea Pigs*. (Routledge and Kegan Paul. London, 1967).

CHAPTER THREE

Drugs[1]

Science's incursion into medicine as described so far has revolution-ised methods of investigation and has thereby improved diagnosis; it has also transformed treatment in surgery. The advances in the treatment of medical conditions, in this century equally astonishing, have also been science-based. They have come from the development of an armoury of new drugs produced by a new industry and assessed for efficacy by scientific methods.

If the man-in-the-street were asked to name the most important change in medicine in this century he would probably say "drugs"; if in this word he included vaccines, toxoids and antitoxins produced by the pharmaceutical industry, as well as the spate of therapeutic drugs, the expert would be inclined to agree. Modern man's new-found confidence that he can control his environment rests in large part on the startling successes of therapeutic and preventive medicine. If he could succeed in controlling his fertility and his aggression (in-cluding his self-destructive urges) the outlook would be bright indeed.

As an *hors d'oeuvre* and as an example of the kind of fact on which this confidence is based a comparison is illuminating. A couple planning in 1900 to have a child had to reckon on an appreciable risk of the mother dying in childbirth (in 1900 the maternal mortality rate in England was 4·81/1,000 total births), and with the probability of one child in seven, even if it were born alive, dying before it was a year old. Today only two mothers in 10,000 die in childbirth and not quite one child in fifty dies in its first year of life. Forty years ago, for every person who today dies from some infectious disease in the first half of life, sixty people succumbed—mainly to whooping-cough, measles, diphtheria or tuberculosis.

The contrast is extreme; the credit side must be acknowledged, and expounded. This is all the more necessary because in recent years medicine and society have been so preoccupied with the debits— drug side-effects, drug-induced diseases, drugs-pejorative, drug costs,

[1] For drug dependence (addiction) see Chapter 10, pp. 210–219.

and even drugs that are too successful because they can prolong life too far. There are signs that the stream of new drugs is starting to dry up. It may soon be possible, therefore, to put the drug explosion in perspective. The middle decades of this century may well be seen as a period in which, although the community benefited enormously from therapeutics, it was exposed to new and unexpected risks, and a period which tested the adaptability and wisdom of the medical profession severely.

The Credit Side

To establish this it is necessary to go back to the turn of the century. Only the very old can remember what medicine was like then; for the rest the contrast between then and now is blurred in our imagination by the brilliance of the scientific revolution that has intervened, a brilliance that has made the earlier period dark and unreal.

The decades around 1900 were a time of famous diagnosticians. The cynic could reasonably say that this was not surprising. There was no other way in which an able doctor could express himself because there were so few remedies for any disease. A quotation from an old text-book of 1901 on the treatment of scarlet fever makes curious reading today.[1] (This disease, together with erysipelas, killed 5,000 people in England and Wales in 1900.)

"In mild cases little is needed beyond careful isolation and free diluents. Tepid baths and sponging the surface are grateful in almost every case. When the temperature is high we must check it by cold sponging, wet packs, rubbing with ice or cold baths ... In severe cases ... the patient must be fed by the nose ... by inserting a small glass funnel ... into the opening of one nostril, closing the other, and pouring egg, beef tea, or other fluid nourishment into the pharynx ... As soon as the eruption is fully out, the whole surface should be anointed with carbolic oil ... great care should be taken during the stage of peeling to keep the patient from draughts. The body should be clothed in flannel ... During convalescence tincture of steel is the most useful drug, and port wine the best form of stimulant when it is required."

Will some of our present ways of treating diseases for which there is no specific remedy strike the same note of futility in another sixty years, or, worse, will they be seen as positively harmful?

[1] Fagge, C. H. and Pye-Smith, P. H. *Textbook of Medicine*. (J. and A. Churchill. London, 4th edn. 1901).

Nowadays, to repeat, the possibility of a wife dying in childbirth, of a child not surviving to adult life, except perhaps as a result of a road accident, hardly crosses a parent's mind. People do not now expect to get serious infectious illnesses, or, if they do, they expect to be cured. This confidence applies, too, to many of the non-infectious diseases and it marks a profound change in the attitude of the patient to his doctor. Kindliness, comforting, a manner radiating confidence, and—reminiscent of the quotation above—advice about bland diet, adequate warmth, and ventilation are no longer enough. Patients expect and demand more positive measures and, thanks to the mass media, as often as not they know broadly what the action should be. In some respects the old sufferer-healer relationship has given place to something more commercial, although most patients are too polite to say so.

The revolution in therapeutics and preventive medicine has come upon us very fast, but already the changed pattern of disease, and this altered attitude to illness, seem very much a part of present day life. Most people who are old enough to remember what things used to be like, say, forty years ago seldom do so: the wards of fever hospitals; the sentence of perhaps life-long invalidism that a diagnosis of pulmonary tuberculosis entailed; young children blue and exhausted from a paroxysm of whooping cough; a child of twelve dying from heart failure a fortnight after his attack of diphtheria began; and the inevitable death of anyone who developed tuberculous meningitis. Perhaps one prefers to forget. What exactly has happened and how has it been achieved?

At the end of the nineteenth century the physician and surgeon had only an exceedingly limited list of effective drugs in his dispensary: nitrous oxide, ether and chloroform as aids to the surgeon; opium and morphine for the relief of pain; digitalis for use in heart failure; and really the only specific remedy—quinine for malaria. This was about all, though perhaps one should mention bromide in the control of epilepsy and the neuroses. The public health authorities' weapons included the general measures of hygiene, sanitation and quarantine which had been so successful in eradicating cholera, and vaccination against smallpox.

The introduction of aspirin in 1899 by Dreser in Germany heralded the pharmaceutical era in which we are still living. The bewildering array of drugs introduced since then can only be summarised briefly and incompletely but even so is formidable enough. The list must include: the barbiturates; the local anaesthetics; vitamins including vitamin B^{12} for pernicious anaemia; vaccines against typhoid, whooping cough, poliomyelitis and measles; antitoxins; toxoids against diphtheria and tetanus; the hormones beginning with insulin and continuing with thyroid, pituitary, adrenal cortical, and sex hormones; the synthetic antimalarials; new general anaesthetics; sulphonamides; antibiotics including the antituberculous drugs; antihypertensives, antihistamines, anticoagulants; the new diuretics; antipsychotic drugs such as chlorpromazine, and the antidepressants.

Reasonably effective remedies are lacking only for the degenerative diseases of arteries, joints and brain, for nearly all virus infections, for most forms of cancer, for chronic bronchitis, for many diseases of the nervous system and for the neuroses. The search for new ones continues and until fairly recently the American drug industry was bringing into the market 400 new drugs or combinations of older drugs each year.[1]

At the close of the nineteenth century pharmacology as a science had hardly begun. Drugs were used empirically because they worked or were supposed to work. In this century advances in physiology, biochemistry and pharmacology have gone hand in hand with the development of new groups of drugs. Each branch of knowledge has fertilised the others and led to new concepts of the nature of disease processes and new theories about how drugs work. To some extent new drugs can be designed for a specific purpose.

The most impressive and immediately obvious results have been in the field of infectious disease. Raw figures of numbers of deaths in England and Wales have been used rather than death rates and one should remember that the reductions in deaths have happened in spite of a rising population. No doubt a similar table giving deaths from infectious diseases in every advanced country in the world would match this one.

These illnesses mainly attack children and young adults, although the age at which people die of tuberculosis has lately increased. This select group of illnesses caused the death in 1925 of 58,000 children and young people. By 1967 the figure had fallen to about 2,300, of whom only 147 were under thirty years old.

Chart I (p. 45) shows the dramatic fall which has occurred in the mortality from all infectious diseases in the *first half of life*.

Many general factors—improved nutrition and reduction of over-crowding for example—must have contributed to the fall in deaths as well as the more obviously medical measures—the use of drugs and campaigns for mass immunisation—and it is impossible to disentangle

[1] Baehr, G. in *Drugs in Our Society*. Ed. Talalay, P. (Johns Hopkins Press, Baltimore, Md. and Oxford University Press. London, 1964).

TABLE 1

Deaths from certain infectious diseases England and Wales

	1925	1930	1935	1940	1945	1950	1955	1960	1965
Scarlet Fever and Erysipelas	1,838	1,774	1,633	365	201	74	15	7	12
Whooping Cough	6,058	2,037	1,584	678	689	394	87	37	21
Diphtheria	2,774	3,497	3,488	2,466	694	49	12	5	0
Measles	5,337	4,188	1,346	855	728	221	174	31	115
Puerperal Sepsis	1,110	1,244	1,006	194	76	21	13	7	4
Meningoccal Infection	354	632	617	2,459	527	283	205	95	112
Typhoid and Paratyphoid	388	313	174	127	44	16	14	3	8
Tetanus	159	133	128	109	79	71	33	18	21
Tuberculosis-all forms	40,392	35,750	29,201	27,871	23,468	15,969	6,492	3,435	2,282
Pulmonary	32,382	29,414	24,603	23,470	19,668	14,077	5,474	2,863	1,844
Meningitis	3,035	2,472	1,847	1,851	1,772	890	132	61	44
Poliomyelitis	156	164	145	159	126	734	241	23	3
Population	38·9m	39·8m	40·6m	41·8m	42·6m	43·8m	44·6m	45·8m	47·9m

Source: Registrar General's Statistical Review for various years—part I Tables, medical—esp. Table 7

the importance of each. One must be cautious about a *post hoc, ergo propter hoc* argument, but it is plain from Table I that deaths from streptococcal infections—scarlet fever, erysipelas, and puerperal sepsis—in that list of diseases were reduced to one-fifth in the quinquennium following the introduction of sulphonamide drugs in 1935; that deaths from diphtheria fell rapidly after the immunisation programme began in 1940; that the largest fall in deaths from tuberculosis took place in the decade 1945–55 after the discovery of streptomycin; and that deaths each year from poliomyelitis were greatly reduced in the years following the mass vaccination campaign which began in 1956.

Deaths from infectious diseases, ages 0-44   Chart I

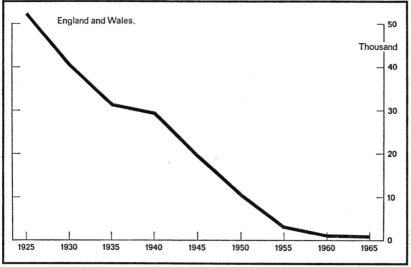

Source: Registrar General's Statistical Reviews. Table 17

The figures speak for themselves. Nevertheless some diseases are subject to inexplicable variations in prevalence and severity and some micro-organisms undergo curious fluctuations in virulence. Epidemic encephalitis (encephalitis lethargica), for example, appeared as a new disease in 1917 and reached epidemic proportions in several of the years between then and 1926. Since that year it has disappeared, at least as an epidemic disease and perhaps, some say, altogether. The virulence of the streptococcus of scarlet fever and the case mortality had been diminishing for many years before the introduction of the sulphonamide drugs. One paediatrician says that the case-mortality had dropped from 13·5% to less than 1% over the

previous fifty years.[1] Diphtheria, too, seems to have undergone
strange fluctuations in prevalence. In 1935 there were about 65,000
notifications and 3,500 deaths from the disease. Yet the eminent and
very trustworthy Sir John Simon writing in 1858 said, "diphtheria is
a disease which, though it was experienced in former times, is well-
nigh unknown to the existing generation of British medical practitioners."[2] Despite these cautions it is probably safe to conclude that
by far the greatest part of the fall in the number of deaths from these
infectious diseases has been due to positive measures of prevention
and treatment.

Some infectious illnesses like diphtheria and whooping cough are
kill-or-cure, others like scarlet fever leave sequels which may kill
later. The near-elimination of deaths from infectious illness, and
efficient treatment to make complications less frequent and severe,
have meant that far larger numbers of people survive at least into
middle life and swell the numbers of the working population. This is
perhaps most strikingly shown in the case of pulmonary tuberculosis:

TABLE 2

Deaths from pulmonary tuberculosis at different ages.
England and Wales.

Year	Under 20	20–29	30–39	40–49	50–59	60 and over
1930	3,769	7,673	5,852	5,290	4,276	2,554
1950	564	2,451	2,422	2,627	2,760	3,253
1955	50	382	740	904	1,277	2,121
1960	17	42	249	372	627	1,556
1965	9	16	64	219	349	1,187

Source: Registrar General's Statistical Reviews.
Part I. Table 17.

Death from this disease, formerly most frequent in the twenties
age group, is now postponed to late middle and old age. Though
the illness can sometimes not be cured, a full working life is usually
possible and the ravages of the disease in early adult life are a thing
of the past.

To a lesser extent the same is true of that most chronic of common
diseases, diabetes mellitus:

[1] Sheldon, W. *Diseases of Infancy and Childhood.* (J. and A. Churchill. London. 5th edn.
1946).
[2] Thomson, D. (1951), *Monthly Bulletin of the Ministry of Health*, 10, 132.

TABLE 3

Deaths from diabetes at various ages.
England and Wales.

Year	Under 15	15–24	25–34	35–44	45–54	55–64	65–74	75+	Total
1900	107	226	245	253	461	690	577	208	2,767
1920	141	247	277	313	483	899	1,012	377	3,749
1930	98	150	202	232	549	1,497	1,990	943	5,661
1950	38	45	76	102	216	592	1,438	1,178	3,685
1955	25	25	59	81	175	547	1,173	1,206	3,290
1960	26	24	49	87	156	577	1,192	1,449	3,560
1965	24	22	46	101	191	632	1,411	1,779	4,206

Source: Registrar General's Statistical Reviews. Part I. Table 17.

But the picture presented by this table is less striking than in the case of pulmonary tuberculosis. Diabetes is mainly a genetically determined disease, and the proportion of the population developing it at any age remains roughly constant. Thus, in a population that has grown by almost 50% since 1900, the number of cases is bound to have increased, even without the improvement in diagnosis that took place in the 1920s. Since then, as with tuberculosis, treatment has postponed the peak age of death from diabetes until the late sixties and seventies, though it should be remembered that, as with any chronic illness, if patients are enabled to live for decades, particularly till they are over sixty, the chance that they will die of some other illness greatly increases.

A host of other illnesses too numerous to mention can today be treated more or less effectively so that the patient can still work, or at least so that death from the illness is postponed or avoided altogether. It is too early yet for the successful onslaught on the infectious diseases to have played much part in swelling the numbers of elderly in the population, but the effect is bound to be seen in the future. Already, of course, the use of antibiotics in the chest infections of the elderly must have given many thousands of people years more of life, even if sometimes this extension is burdensome.

The credit side of the drugs revolution, therefore, is well established. How has this success been achieved?

Where Drugs Come From

The answer seems self-evident: the pharmaceutical industry—and in the sense that it does in fact manufacture and market these potent and life-saving drugs the answer is correct. It also makes most of the vaccines, antitoxins and toxoids used in preventive medicine. But who discovered the drug in naturally occurring materials? Who purified it? Who tested it on animals to define its physiological and therapeutic possibilities and its toxicity? Who altered its molecule and made it less toxic and more effective? Who thought out the steps in large-scale manufacture? Who altered the conditions at one stage so that the yield was greatly increased? Who synthesised drugs from simple materials? There are no simple answers to these questions and they have been different for different groups of drugs. It is false to think that drug discoveries have been made by pure scientists working in universities or in government research institutes, that the basic research on defining the properties and toxicity of a drug has continued there on small quantities produced on a laboratory bench in glassware, and that after the publication of promising results in a paper or two in a learned journal a drug company becomes interested and starts large scale manufacture. Such a picture has been true in respect of only a small proportion of the drugs discovered in this century. Since the end of the Second World War it has become plain that the newer major discoveries are more often made in the research laboratories of the pharmaceutical industry itself, and most vaccine research is carried out there as well.

Professor Ernst Chain, who with Lord Florey and others helped to develop penicillin, gave a lecture[1] in 1963 in which he analysed the relative contribution of academic institutions and of industry to research in drugs. He described in detail the history of the discovery and development of many different drugs and firmly concluded that the closest collaboration between industry and the universities and research institutes is the surest road to success.

Pure research is supposed to have unimpeachable lily-white motives. In a society that reveres the academic the singleminded search for new knowledge is a high and very respectable motive. But wholly disinterested people are rare and certainly in medical research other motives operate as well, though few would go so far as to patent a lucky discovery and sell it to a drug firm—which, however, is not entirely unknown. The impure motives are less base than this: pure research can be a quiet and comfortable life and one can be left for long periods to one's own devices without much pressure for results; a piece of research may be undertaken almost solely to yield an M.D. or a B.Sc.; or a lucky break can lead to fame, demands for lectures, and a pleasant increase in amour-propre.

Many of our drugs have certainly been the outcome of pure research—notably the vitamins, from the germ of the idea with Hopkins and with Funk in the early years of the century, to their isolation and ultimate synthesis a quarter of a century later; insulin, the antihistamines, penicillin, and stilboestrol had similar origins.

Many other drugs have been the outcome of more obviously commercial motives, though the use of this word does not imply a moral judgment. The account which follows makes use of Professor Chain's material but is mainly derived from other sources.[2] [3] [4] [5]

The pharmaceutical industry as we know it began at the turn of

[1] Chain, E. B. (1963), *Nature*, **200,** 441.
[2] Salter, W. T. *Textbook of Pharmacology.* (W. B. Saunders. Philadelphia and London 1952).
[3] Goodman, L. S. and Gilman, A. *The Pharmacological Basis of Therapeutics.* (Macmillan. New York, 1955).
[4] Appelzweig, N. *Steroid Drugs.* (McGraw Hill. New York and London, 1962).
[5] *Drugs in Our Society.*

D

the century in Germany as an off-shoot of the dyestuffs section of
the chemical industry and Temkin[1] quotes a remark of Buchheim at
that time which foreshadows many current troubles:

"The chemical industry of our days produces various substances
for which no market can as yet be found. Under these circumstances,
the idea suggests itself that it might be possible to use these products
as drugs. We know that a great number of physicians, without rhyme
or reason, go after every new remedy that is presented to them. If an
industrialist is but shrewd enough to advertise sufficiently, he usually
succeeds in increasing the sale of his product—for some time at
least—and thus enriching himself."

The by-products were aspirin and the other antipyretics and
eventually the sulphonamides and the oral antidiabetic drugs.
Many other groups of drugs, the barbiturates and the organic
arsenicals used in the treatment of syphilis and some tropical
diseases, for example, were discovered and developed by this pharmaceutical offspring of the chemical industry in Germany. The
search for new drugs yielding more profit and, of course, helping
diseased mankind reached, from time to time, a kind of frenzy as
chemists played about with molecules, introducing a methyl group
here or altering a side chain there. Since barbitone was synthesised
by Fischer and von Mehring and introduced to medicine in 1903,
and since phenobarbitone was discovered by several chemists in 1912,
2,500 barbiturates[2] have been synthesised and assessed and fifty have
been marketed for clinical use. The sulphonamides, the antihistamines and the phenothiazine antipsychotic drugs are other examples
of groups of compounds that have been subjected in the hands of
chemists of many countries to this intensive kind of manipulation.

It is very costly indeed, but very rewarding for the firm that discovers the best of the group. It is also very precarious. A company's
considerable investment in doing the basic research of a new drug,
in manufacture, testing and marketing may, according to a recent
estimate, amount to £2 million. A minimum figure of £200,000 has
been mentioned. Sums of this order may be lost if a rival discovers
a better drug of the same group, or if a wholly new group of drugs is
discovered with superior qualities in treating the same illness. A
large investment in producing antistreptococcal and antistaphyl-
ococcal sera was lost, for example, when the first sulphonamide was
introduced in 1936, and it is said that Lederle spent $13 million on

[1] *Drugs in Our Society.*
[2] Bogue, Y. *The Times*, 25 February, 1965.

poliomyelitis vaccine research but, with the ultimate success of Sabin's oral live vaccine, lost most of it.[1] Severe losses can occur, too, if a dissatisfied employee with sufficient knowledge, or a spy, transmits information to a rival. This has happened to one of the original manufacturers of a tetracycline drug.

To the protection that patent law offers in many countries the big drug firms who do research and development have understandably added stringed security measures, fences, passes and all-but-armed guards.

A further motive, a hope of political advantage or a fear of being caught at a disadvantage in wartime, has sometimes lain behind a very expensive programme of research. During the 1920s the German pharmaceutical industry conducted a frenzied search for synthetic antimalarial drugs more effective than quinine. More than 12,000 compounds were prepared and tested culminating in the discovery of plasmoquin and mepacrine. In 1941 the United States was cut off from most of its supplies of quinine and its industry had quickly to master the problems of producing mepacrine. It did so, but the drawbacks of this drug encouraged an intense search for a more successful antimalarial drug. Hundreds of products, again, were synthesised and tested and the result was the introduction of chloroquine. The war also gave a great fillip to steroid research. It was erroneously reported that German airmen were being given an adrenal hormone to protect them from the effects of high altitudes. Not to be outdone, an American drug company, on official suggestion, carried out an expensive programme of research, which resulted eventually in the discovery of cortisone. The effects of this drug on rheumatoid arthritis and other diseases were completely unexpected, and were only found out later.

The list of countries that have produced several worthwhile drugs is short—Germany, France, Switzerland, Great Britain and the United States. All have well developed chemical and pharmaceutical industries, capital to risk for the opportunity of great rewards, a tradition of academic scientific research, and the opportunity for co-operation between "pure" research institutions and industry. Russia, Italy, Japan and the countries of Northern and Eastern Europe are missing from the list. In the case of the Communist countries, at least, it may well be that because they disregard the patents of others they have no need to compete. They can pirate the inventions of other people by reading the world's scientific literature, or by paying for inside information.

[1] Wilson, J. R. *Margin of Safety.* (Collins. London, 1963).

Cancer, virus and degenerative diseases are still in the main untreatable. It is very important indeed that research into new drugs should continue. The thrusting, high-risk, pharmaceutical industry has been accused, particularly in the United States where most research is undertaken and most discovery now is made, of serious abuses. Setting them right should not cause injury to the goose that lays such golden eggs. To judge whether injury is being done the abuses must first be specified and the remedial action taken or in prospect set out.

Criticisms of the Pharmaceutical Industry

In the last ten years or so the drug industry, especially in the United States, has come in for heavy criticism. It has been accused of a variety of abuses—excessive prices and profits, immoral marketing methods, misdirected research, inflated claims and the playing-down of side-effects.

From its origins in the extraction of medicinal products from plants and as a by-product of the chemical industry the pharmaceutical industry has developed with almost explosive violence. It is now very big business indeed. The American Pharmaceutical Manufacturers Association has estimated that the sales of ethical[1] pharmaceuticals in 1965 amounted to $4,210 million ; $365 million was spent on research and development in 1965. In Britain the industry since the war has been invaded by foreign firms, mainly American and Swiss. American firms account now for half the sales and the British share has been reduced to a quarter.[2] Total output in 1966 was £308 million and it has doubled in the last eight years. The industry's expenditure on research in 1966 was £13 million. The industry in Britain has become a significant exporter; in 1966 excess of exports over imports [3] totalled £56 million.[4] Although the industry in the United States dwarfs the British, growth and high research costs are features of both.

A common and frequently justified criticism of the drug industry is that its prices are too high. Everyone agrees that drug firms pursue a risky business and that they should be able to recoup their costs and the price of their expensive failures. But, after a successful drug has

[1] Drugs not advertised directly to the public.
[2] *The Times*. 15 December, 1967.
[3] The Sainsbury Committee has produced a much more cautious net figure computed on a basis different from the industry's more flattering estimate. See *Report of the Committee of Enquiry into the relationship of the Pharmaceutical Industry with the National Health Service 1965–1967* (The Sainsbury Committee). (H.M.S.O. London, 1967). Table 19.
[4] *The Pharmaceutical Industry and the Nation's Health*. A.B.P.I. September, 1967.

been on the market for three or four years, the price should begin to come down. The price of penicillin, for example, fell by 90% between 1943 and 1950 as did that of streptomycin between 1948 and 1955. In the case of the tetracyclines, however, the price in America remained at 50 cents a capsule between 1948 and 1957. In 1968 in Britain the cost of tetracyclines from American sources was still ninepence a capsule even though, for many years, it has cost only three-halfpence to produce.

Criticisms are also made of tacit agreements between drug firms to keep prices up, the crushing of small firms that sell at lower prices, and excessive profit-taking. In the United States there has been a collision between three large drug firms and antitrust legislation in which the companies have been expensively worsted.

Marketing methods have also come in for criticism. According to the Kefauver enquiry the U.S. drug industry in 1959–60 was spending $750 millions a year on promotion. This was 24% of sales, a proportion twice as high as in any other industry. In Britain the industry in 1965 spent £15·4 million or 13·9% of sales.[1]

As a growth industry drugs have an essential weakness. The industry uses the sales methods of the mid-twentieth century, which may well be appropriate to a growing consumer market but not to a market that shrinks, or remains stable, if the industry's products are successful. People can be persuaded to buy a chicken for every pot, two cars for every garage and a new and better washing machine every year. But the demand for drugs is naturally limited by the amount of sickness in the population, however much the industry tries to widen the definition of sickness. Thus, the amount of polio vaccine needed in Britain is limited by the number of babies born each year. As the American industry's representative said to the Kefauver Committee[2] "We can't put two sick people in every bed where there is only one person sick."

Most of the promotion money goes on trying to persuade doctors, who are in fact whether they like it or not the retailers, to prescribe a particular proprietary brand. As one American writer[3] has put it, ". . . perhaps no other group in the country is so insistently sought after, chased, wooed, pressured, and downright importuned." The cost to the drug companies worked out at $4,000 for each doctor and each doctor received 4,000 promotional pieces each year. In Britain the pressure is less intense, but the drug firms spend £250 on

[1] The Sainsbury Committee.

[2] U.S. Congress, Senate, *Subcommittee on Antitrust and Monopoly.* (1961), Report 448. p. 157. Quoted in *Drugs in Our Society.*

[3] Garai, P. R. in *Drugs in Our Society*, p. 191.

each doctor for their "representatives" (detail men) and this amount is only 45 % of their total expenditure on sales promotion.[1] Each general practitioner in addition receives an average of seven pieces of mail a day, as well as being subject to other forms of pressure—advertising in the medical and paramedical press, free samples, minor presents (desk pads and calendars), and the financing of clinical trials.

Persuasion is all the easier because the doctors do not foot the bill. No doubt long years of training, in which a respect for scientific method and a sceptical attitude should have been implanted, ought to have produced a resistance to these methods; but the sheer weight of persuasion and the playing upon that Achilles' heel of professional men, the fear of being out of date, is often enough to undermine caution. It is all too easy to pull out the prescription pad and hand out quantities of the latest tranquilliser, antibiotic or diuretic under its memorable brand name—to give examples: Librium, Saluric, Stelazine, Naclex—than to think of the often very unmemorable generic name—chlordiazepoxide, chlorothiazide, trifluperazine, hydroflumethiazide—and it is sometimes alleged that drug firms deliberately design the generic name to be a tongue twister. It is more difficult still to sit back and to reflect on whether the patient needs any drug at all and on whether there is any hard evidence that the prescribed drug does what it is supposed to do.

So long as doctors still prescribe one brand of oxytetracycline which is more than three times the price of another, and paracetamol which when branded costs almost twice as much as when unbranded, firms will continue to spend huge sums on promotion. In Britain the drug bill to the taxpayer and in America to the patient will therefore continue to be much bigger than it need be.

The excesses, both of price and publicity, that have evoked so much criticism of late recall an earlier epoch when it was the methods of the other half of the industry that were under attack. In 1909 the British Medical Association published *Secret Remedies*, an analysis of the ingredients and cost of some hundreds of proprietary cures and of the claims made for them. This and the companion volume *More Secret Remedies* (1912) proved to be bestsellers and sold more than 100,000 copies. Some of the remedies, like Pomie's Anticataract Mixture, Tuberculozyne, and Dill's Diabetic Mixture, do not seem to have stayed the course. Others are still familiar. Phosferine at that time contained quinine, sulphuric and phosphoric acid and alcohol—the formula may have been changed since. It claimed to be a proven remedy for a long list of disorders including

[1] The Sainsbury Committee.

that vanished condition "brain fag". The estimated cost of the ingredients was ½d. and the retail price (including tax and packaging) 2s. 9d.—a mark-up, to use the current phrase, of 6,000%. Beecham's Pills at that time contained aloes, ginger and soap. The price without tax was about a hundred times the cost of the ingredients.

Complaints of excessive mark-ups have a familiar ring today. So do these words from the 1912 volume:

"Some employ big posters on hoardings, others—an increasing number—have fringed the chief railway lines of the country with great boards bearing the names of their nostrums; almost all agree in making large use of newspapers, magazines and other periodicals, and of copious distribution, through various agencies, of circulars and pamphlets . . . In the case of another nostrum, a single article, which was before the courts a few years ago, it was proved in evidence that in five years 83 million pamphlets had been issued, and that, in the words of the judge 'they had flooded the English-speaking world with their advertisements'."

At least it can be said of the patent medicines that only a few were positively harmful unlike some of the nostrums sold on the American market before the passing of the Pure Food and Drugs Act of 1906,[1] which contained opiates.

Research methods are also open to criticism. No one denies that the results of the bulk of American pharmaceutical research have been brilliant. The criticism is that a proportion of it is misdirected. As Professor Gaddum[2] has said, "it is often possible for a chemist and a pharmacologist working together to test the effect of minor changes in the molecular structure of a drug and so gradually to increase its potency till, after a few years, they have a molecule which is ten or one hundred times more active than the original drug."

This wizardry, and the discovery of new groups of drugs, are the rosy aspect which the companies in their own defence like to dwell on and which the public accepts as justifying high profits. But according to another professor of pharmacology,[3] the purpose of much of the work done by American drug firms is partly to exploit and market products originating abroad but "mostly to modify the original drug just enough to get a patentable derivative". Molecular manipulation has these two meanings.

A favourite device, though this can hardly be called research, is to

[1] Young, J. H. *The Toadstool Millionaires.* (Princeton University Press. Princeton, N.J. 1961).
[2] *Drugs in Our Society.*
[3] Meyers, F. H. quoted in *The New Yorker.* 21 March, 1964.

give a new name to a combination of existing drugs and then to turn on the whole blaring orchestra of publicity to convince the doctor that this freshly coloured tablet is a new drug, or that the two or more constituents act "synergistically"—implying that the total effect of the combination is greater than the sum of the effects of each constituent acting alone.

A further criticism of research methods is that some drugs are issued and marketed after quite insufficient clinical study. In general this charge cannot be levelled at the large drug firms, which make very great efforts, both in their own laboratories and in the clinical field, to satisfy themselves of the safety and usefulness of their drug. They have too much at stake to risk disasters and on many occasions, as a safeguard, have limited the supply of a new drug for some time to hospitals only.

The drug industry can also be charged with making excessive claims and neglecting side-effects. This is a charge which sticks, as anyone will know who has talked to firms' representatives. The side-effects referred to here are the immediate and known ones and not those long-term unknown ones such as were responsible for the withdrawal of thalidomide. The dangers of such a head in the sand policy are two-fold: first, if a drug is publicised as harmless it will be widely used for trivial complaints, and if it is an antibiotic its future usefulness in serious infections will be jeopardised because the growth of resistant strains of micro-organisms will have been encouraged; second, doctors will tend to use the drugs heedlessly and a crop of side-effects, some of them serious, will injure not only some patients but also the drug's reputation and sales. It may be years before the balance between a drug's usefulness and its liability to poison is struck. This happened with chloramphenicol and with one of the oral antidiabetic drugs.

Perhaps one cannot do better as a summary of the pros and cons of pharmaceutical developments in this century than to quote President Kennedy:[1]

"The successful development of more than 9,000 new drugs in the last 25 years has saved countless lives and relieved millions of victims of acute and chronic illnesses. However, the new drugs are being placed on the market with no requirements that there be either advance proof that they will be effective . . . or the prompt reporting of adverse reactions. These new drugs present greater hazards as well as greater potential benefits than ever before—for they are

Kennedy, J. F. *Message on Consumer Protection.* 1962. Quoted in *Drugs in Our Society.*

widely used, they are often very potent and they are promoted by aggressive sales campaigns that may tend to overstate their merits and fail to indicate the risks involved in their use."

Control of the Pharmaceutical Industry

The criticisms of the pharmaceutical industry, like those of the patent medicine trade fifty years ago, have provoked different measures in different countries. In the United States, where private enterprise medicine flourishes, government control over the drug industry came earlier than in Britain, perhaps because in a highly competitive country the excesses of the industry, excessive claims on behalf of a drug and excessive measures to market it, became apparent more quickly. Whatever the reason, in 1962, the year when the thalidomide disaster came to light in Britain, and prompted the British Government to take the first step towards safety control, some at least of the findings of the Kefauver enquiry were given legislative form in America.

The Kefauver-Harris Drug Amendments carried the existing responsibility of the American Government as overseer a big step forward. Government control now takes three main forms. First, the Food and Drug Administration has to be notified before a drug is submitted to clinical investigation and has to be informed of the progress of the investigation so that the trial can be called off if the drug proves unsafe or ineffective. Secondly, much greater emphasis is laid on the effectiveness of a new drug, which cannot be marketed unless there is "substantial evidence", as shown by the number and quality of the investigations, to support the claims made on its behalf. Thirdly, in the advertising of a drug to the medical profession, its promoters must include, besides a reasonable claim of what it can do, a summary of its limitations, contra-indications and side-effects.[1]

Senator Kefauver had also been concerned about the high price of new drugs. But he failed in his attempt to have the patent law amended so that after a time prices would come down. Although this frontal attack on patent rights failed, they are under attack from the side. A leading manufacturer has complained[2] that patents arising out of any discoveries in the drug field made with the help of scientists aided by Government grants remain with the Government. New products, therefore, cannot be patented by firms if Government-aided scientists have played even the smallest part in their discovery

---

[1] Goodrich, W. W. in *Drugs in Our Society.* p. 141 ff.
[2] Connor, J. T. op. cit. p. 117 ff.

or development. This policy may well lower prices, but it could be disastrous if it undermines co-operation between academic research institutes and the industry.

In Britain until 1962, the Ministry of Health, faced with the rising cost of drugs in the national health service, was more concerned with prices than with safety, even though, by comparison with the United States and most other Western countries, expenditure per head on drugs is low. The Ministry followed up its voluntary price agreement with the industry, which had been in force since 1957, by invoking in 1961 a section of the Patents Act that allowed it to use a patented invention for Crown use; as it owned the hospitals of the health service it tendered for the supply of some drugs and was able to obtain them from abroad at much lower prices than the patentees were asking. Pfizer's, the manufacturers of oxytetracycline, retorted by bringing a legal action that was fought, up to the House of Lords, and finally lost by the company. In the meantime, the thalidomide tragedy, and the pressure of public opinion following it, stirred the Ministry of Health into a concern for safety as well as for costs.

At first, this concern, in which the medical profession and the drug industry shared, expressed itself in the establishment of a voluntary body, the Dunlop Committee, in 1964. The committee lacked penal sanctions and, as in America, the responsibility for testing a drug was left with the manufacturers; but the committee examined every drug submitted to it for toxicity, efficacy and evidence of adequate clinical trials, and its power to inform every doctor of the danger of prescribing a drug not submitted to its scrutiny guaranteed co-operation from the industry. At the same time doctors were asked to send the committee instances of unusual or hitherto unreported side-effects. In its four years of existence the committee issued only a handful of pamphlets to doctors about adverse reactions, but much more work goes on behind the scenes. In 1965 the committee considered submissions from manufacturers to conduct clinical trials on or to market 1,041 drugs,[1] and it received from doctors more than 4,000 reports of suspected adverse reactions to drugs in use.

Despite some American expert opinion that the quick, economical and voluntary Dunlop Committee had advantages over the FDA's more rigid methods, the procedure was replaced in 1968 by a statutory one. An official Medicines Commission was set up to license the manufacture and marketing of drugs for human and veterinary use, to supervise their safety, quality and efficacy and to ensure that

[1] *Annual Report of the Committee on Safety of Drugs* (The Dunlop Committee). (H.M.S.O. London, 1966).

promotional material is accurate. The commission is not independent of the Government, as was recommended by the Sainsbury Committee on the drug industry, which had been set up in 1965 and reported in the autumn of 1967. On the other hand, the new legislation does not go so far as the Sainsbury Committee would have liked in respect of drug prices: it does not, that is, ensure that the price of drugs is brought to doctors' notice; and it does not abolish brand names for new products.

Thus, both America and Britain, with their very different, in fact opposing, types of medical care, have reached virtually the same stage in their governments' efforts to control the industry that has so revolutionised medical care. Both governments have failed to make any real breach in patent law and the use of brand names, and drug prices remain higher than they should be in both countries. On the other hand, the British Government has now caught up with the American in assuming responsibility for safety, efficacy and honesty. It still has to be seen whether these virtues are being attained at the expense of the industry's pushful initiative and enterprise: the goose may well go broody.

There have been other changes in the last few years in addition to legislative action. For instance, in 1966 the British industry revised its code of marketing practice in response to criticisms; it seems also to have altered its method of approach to doctors. In the last year or two the spate of promotional material arriving through doctors' letter-boxes has become a trickle. Instead, free periodicals full of informed authoritative articles arrive. Though financed by the drug advertising they carry, these magazines seem unbiased. Their independence from pressure is no doubt guaranteed by the high standing of their editors and advisory committees.

As postgraduate education for doctors who qualified long ago these journals and their official and professional companions have been supplemented by other means—by refresher courses, for example. But perhaps the most significant step forward has been the opening of medical centres in many hospitals where general practitioners can meet their specialist colleagues informally. In this setting the virtues and vices of new drugs, in particular their side-effects, are very common topics of conversation.

Side-effects and Toxicity

Many people maintain that it is only in the last fifteen years or so that the side-effects of drugs have become a familiar problem. The earlier discoveries of drugs such as aspirin, the vitamins, liver extract, insulin and even penicillin seemed to be innocuous even if they were occasionally wrongly used. There is some truth in this, and it is indeed only very recently that groups of drugs have been used which as often as not have dangerous side-effects—the antihypertensive drugs, the corticosteroids, the phenothiazines, the antidepressants the anticoagulants and so forth. But as a general proposition, unpleasant and even dangerous side-effects are not new, and it is only a minority of effective drugs that lacks them. Physicians newly released from therapeutic impotence by the spate of new drugs now find themselves too often in the predicament of the sorcerer's apprentice.

Even such useful and old-fashioned remedies as digitalis, aspirin, quinine and phenacetin are not free from risk. Until recently phenacetin was thought to be the safest of the aniline derivatives and a very useful antipyretic. It was known to be far safer than acetanilid, which years ago was a dangerous ingredient of several proprietary headache pills, or an adulterant in others. It has been known for a long time that excessive doses of phenacetin could cause both cyanosis, because of the conversion of some haemoglobin to methaemoglobin, and a haemolytic anaemia. More recently Swiss workers have discovered[1] that phenacetin is a possible cause of one variety of nephritis. Other people have confirmed that excessive self-medication with phenacetin is much commoner in the history of those with this disease than in controls and that the severity of the illness is greater in those who have taken large amounts of this drug for a long time. The disease becomes less severe if phenacetin is given up. The evidence incriminating the drug is not wholly convincing, but it is accumulating, and there have been confirmatory reports from America and Scotland.[2] The Swedes, the Swiss, and the Danes have been sufficiently impressed to have made phenacetin a prescription drug, and the Pharmaceutical Society in Britain has recommended chemists to warn regular users of the drug of its dangers and to suggest alternatives.

Here is a prime example of one important category of side-effects, those noticed only after a drug has been in use for some years. In the case of phenacetin, although several other side-effects became quickly known, it was more than sixty years before its effect on the kidney was suspected. The serious effects on the eye of the antimalarial drug

[1] Spuhler, O. and Zollinger, H. U. (1953), *Zeitschr. Klin. Med.*, **151**, 1. Referred to in Prescott, L. F. (1966), *Lancet*, **ii**, 1143.
[2] Prescott, L. F. (1966), loc. sit.

chloroquine were described in 1958 and 1959, twelve years after the drug was introduced.[1] [2]

Then there is the intolerance to cheese of some patients who are having mono-amine oxidase inhibitor drugs for depression. This strange, alarming and sometimes dangerous side-effect was first reported in 1963, about four years after the group of drugs was introduced.[3] Since then research has shown just how this side-effect is caused.[4] Cheese, particularly some varieties of mature cheddar, contains quite large amounts of the toxic amine tyramine. Ordinarily this amine is converted by an enzyme, mono-amine oxidase, contained in the lining of the gut and in the liver into the harmless hydroxyphenylacetic acid which is excreted in the urine. Patients being treated for depression with mono-amine oxidase inhibitors can no longer deal with tyramine, which after a cheese meal may accumulate in the body. A small proportion develop an exceedingly severe headache, flushing, palpitation, sweating, and a steep rise in blood pressure. Some deaths have been reported. Three other foodstuffs may also give trouble.[5] [6] The pods of broad beans contain dihydroxyphenylalanine, which is converted in the body into the toxic amine dopamine. Patients who are having mono-amine oxidase inhibitors cannot detoxicate this. Yeast extracts, too, as they contain appreciable amounts of both tyramine and histamine can cause the same unpleasant and potentially dangerous reaction, and bananas, because of their 5-hydroxytryptamine content, also have to be avoided.

By far the most extraordinary case, however, of a familiar drug producing side-effects that are only identified years later is that of pink disease (acrodynia). This is, or perhaps one should now say was, a mysterious disease of young children, who developed disturbances of the nervous system, extreme irritability and a peculiar pinkness of the arms and legs.

The disease was originally described in Australia in 1914,[7] but a similar illness had been described much earlier and had been thought to be a variant of pellagra, known now but not then to be due to a deficiency of nicotinic acid in the diet. The mortality in pink disease was about 5% and even twenty years ago the cause was a complete

[1] Hobbs, H. E. and Calnan, C. D. (1958), *Lancet*, **i,** 1207.
[2] Hobbs, H. E., Sorsby, A. and Freedman, A. (1959), *Lancet*, **ii,** 478.
[3] Blackwell, B. (1963), *Lancet*, **ii,** 414.
[4] Blackwell, B. and Mabbitt, L. A. (1965), *Lancet*, **i,** 938.
[5] Hodge, J. H., Nye, E. R. and Emerson, G. W. (1964), *Lancet*, **i,** 1108.
[6] Blackwell, B., Marley, E. and Mabbitt, L. A. (1965), *Lancet*, **i,** 941.
[7] Swift, H. (1914), Report of Australasian Medical Congress, p. 547, referred to in Dathan, J. G. and Harvey, C. C. (1965) *Brit. Med. J.*, **i,** 1181.

mystery. The theories about the cause of it ranged from an unknown infection to a possible dietary deficiency. It was not until 1945 that two Americans in Cincinnati began to suspect that the disease was a manifestation of mercury intoxication. The illness is uncommon in Ohio, and it was only in 1948 that they were able to publish details of the examination of twenty cases (with controls).[1] All the established cases had been having calomel, the mercury-containing purgative, by mouth or mercury ointment rubbed in the skin, and all were excreting quite large amounts of mercury in their urine. Mercury has been used medicinally at least since the sixteenth century, and its toxic possibilities have long been recognised, but the recognition of this variant twenty years ago by Professors Warkany and Hubbard came about because of the latter's invention of a method of estimating the amount of mercury in the urine. There are still some people who cannot bring themselves to believe that mercury is the only cause of this disease, but they must be finding it difficult not to bow to majority opinion in the face of the most recent figures.[2] In the five years 1950–54 189 deaths occurred from pink disease. In 1954, as a result of the publicity, the manufacturers of teething powders containing mercury withdrew them and in the years of 1959–63 only five children died. Certainly the single death in 1963 was caused by teething powders of the old type bought from a village shop, and many health authorities both before and since have been collecting these forgotten but dangerous packets from shops in their areas.

Only one of the major drug disasters of this century has been of this delay-in-recognition type. Thalidomide was in use as a hypnotic for only a few years until it was withdrawn. But in this time enough women had taken it between the fourth and seventh week of pregnancy to produce over 7,000 babies with deformed limbs. It is extremely difficult to see how this kind of catastrophe can be prevented, for the results of tests in other species may be a quite inadequate guide to what will happen in man. One consequence of this tragedy has been to drive home to the medical profession and to the public more forcefully than any number of admonitions from professors of pharmacology the lesson that new drugs are potent for ill as well as for good. Patients now, for the first time, ask their doctors if some drug proposed for them is safe, and what side-effects are to be expected.

Two of the other major disasters concerned vaccines. In 1928 after seven years of research Professor Calmette introduced BCG, a live attenuated bovine tuberculosis vaccine, to immunise children against

[1] Warkany, J. and Hubbard, D. M. (1948), *Lancet*, **i,** 829.
[2] Dathan, J. G. and Harvey, C. C. (1965). loc. cit.

tuberculosis. Two years later 72 children died at Lübeck because, as was later shown, the vaccine had been improperly prepared locally and was contaminated with a virulent strain of bacillus. Although the use of BCG in France and the Scandinavian countries went ahead, the Lübeck disaster delayed its acceptance in Britain and the United States, and it was not until after the Second World War that it was used in either country on a large scale.

Similarly in the United States in 1955, at the peak of the acclaim that greeted the results of large-scale tests of the Salk killed poliomyelitis vaccine, there were disturbing reports of paralytic poliomyelitis developing in children inoculated with the vaccine prepared by one manufacturer. Altogether 204 cases were reported with 11 deaths, but minor alterations in the technique of manufacture and more rigid testing of batches of prepared vaccine eliminated the risk of live virus surviving. By the next year the immunisation campaign was in full swing again and other countries had regained confidence in the Salk method. This confidence was soon to languish and, despite many years of apprehension of the dangers of disaster from using a live attenuated vaccine, the Sabin live vaccine gradually ousted the Salk over the years 1960–63.

The remaining large-scale catastrophe was of quite a different type. In 1937 a chemist in the United States, in trying to produce a palatable liquid form of the antibacterial drug sulphanilamide, which had recently been discovered in Germany, used diethylene glycol—one variety of antifreeze—as the solvent. Though he did not know it at the time, and later committed suicide, the solvent is highly toxic and 107 people died after taking this "elixir".

But these disasters, dramatic though they may have been, have been responsible for only a small proportion of the deaths which drugs have caused over the years; of course, serious but non-fatal reactions to drugs are far commoner still. The statement refers solely to drugs used therapeutically and excludes accidental poisoning, particularly in children, industrial poisoning, and suicide. An overdose of drugs has now become the second commonest method of suicide.

The literature of drug reactions is by now enormous and they are one of the most common topics for papers in the medical press, conferences, symposia and the like; at least two books have been published about them.[1][2] Adverse reactions have been reported to

[1] Spain, D. M. *The Complications of Modern Medical Practice.* (Grune and Stratton. New York and London, 1963).
[2] Meyler, L. and Peck, H. M. *Drug-induced Diseases.* (Royal Vangorcum. Assen, Netherlands, 1962).

almost every effective drug, and there is a long and growing list of drugs that have been withdrawn or have fallen into disuse because of them: amidopyrine, for example, because of its effect on leucocytes; dihydrostreptomycin because of deafness; and iproniazid for depression because of its liability to damage the liver. Drugs have produced what amount to new diseases; for example, the extreme motor restlessness, never before witnessed, sometimes seen in patients who are being treated for schizophrenia with one of the piperazine antipsychotics such as trifluperazine (Stelazine), and the grave "superinfections" with resistant staphylococci or with yeast-like organisms that may occur after treatment with the tetracycline antibiotics.

Unpleasant or dangerous effects of drugs are not easy to classify, in part because the mechanisms are not fully known in many cases, but the following headings contain most of them with the exception of the separate problem of addiction.

a. Side-effects caused by the pharmacological actions of the drug itself: few drugs act solely on one physiological system and even aspirin used as an antipyretic very often has effects on the stomach. The antidepressants all have atropine-like effects and cause dryness of the mouth and constipation; cortisone produces widespread changes—hypertension, obesity, moon-face, and disturbance of water-balance; both the antihistamine and the antipsychotic phenothiazine drugs produce drowsiness.

b. Overdosage: with many drugs the difference between inadequate and excessive dosage is small and an overdose can easily be given; this may cause bleeding in anticoagulant therapy, collapse and loss of consciousness in patients having hypotensive drugs, and heart-block in people who are given digitalis. Toxic effects from overdosage are particularly likely to occur in those patients whose ability to excrete drugs is impaired by previous damage to their kidneys.

c. Idiosyncrasy: people vary enormously in their tolerance of some drugs both initially, as with chlorpromazine which makes some sleepy in a dose of 75 mg daily and leaves others alert even after 1,000 mg a day, and in the longer term. Insulin, barbiturates and, of course, alcohol are examples of drugs to which tolerance may develop. Some idiosyncrasies have been shown to have a genetic basis expressed in an enzyme-deficiency. The muscle relaxant, suxamethonium, used in anaesthesia occasionally paralyses respiration for a prolonged period. Patients in whom this occurs have been shown to have an abnormally low level of the enzyme pseudocholinesterase in their blood plasma. Similarly people who lack the enzyme glucose-6-dehydrogenase in their blood are intolerant of the anti-malarial primaquine and develop a haemolytic anaemia if it is given to them.

d. Allergy and hypersensitivity reactions: these differ from idiosyncrasy in that the effects bear no relation either to the dose of drug or to its ordinary pharmacological action. The immunity defences of the body are involved, and such symptoms as asthma, skin rashes, vomiting, diarrhoea, loss of consciousness and cardio-vascular collapse develop soon after the drug is given to a sensitised patient. Such reactions are common and vary in severity from the trivial to a fatal anaphylactic shock. A great range of drugs has been known to produce allergic reactions, and unfortunately penicillin, formerly considered so safe, is so liable to evoke skin reactions when applied to the body surface that its external use has been virtually given up. More serious still, anaphylactic reactions to the drug when given by injection or by mouth have become all too common; there are reports that, by 1957, 1,000 fatal reactions to penicillin had been recorded in the United States—a much greater number of deaths than was caused by all the major drug disasters added together.

Accurate figures are hard to come by. Few official reports deal with deaths from drugs. Spain[1] makes the astonishing remark: "It is estimated that upwards of 1,000 deaths annually [sic] may be attri-buted to anaphylactic shock from penicillin." Feinberg[2] is more conservative: "it is reasonable to suppose that 100–300 fatalities from such reactions [penicillin allergy] occur annually in the United States." Meyler and Peck[3] state: "W.H.O. reports that in 1957 some 1,000 fatal reactions to penicillin had been reported in the U.S.A. alone." In England and Wales in 1965 official reports[4] state that penicillin caused three deaths.

It is likely that many of the cases of blood dyscrasias (that is, anaemias and dangerous decreases in the number of white cells, of jaundice and of damage to the liver that are due to such drugs as quinine, barbiturates, pyramidon, sulphapyridine, phenylbutazone, chlorpromazine and chlorpropamide involve immune mechanisms.

It is no surprise that fourteen years ago 50 out of 1,000 in-patients

---

[1] Spain, D. M., op. cit.

[2] Feinberg, S. M. (1961), *J. Amer. med. Ass.*, **159**, 1452.

[3] Meyler, L. and Peck, H. M., op. cit.

[4] *Registrar General's Statistical Review for* 1965. Part III. Commentary. (H.M.S.O. London, 1968).

E

in a large American hospital[1] developed some serious complication, which could only be ascribed to drugs, in the course of their treatment. In 1966, a census of all the patients in a large London general hospital showed that of the 468 patients in residence on a particular day 163 were medical cases. Of these, five had been *admitted* because of some complication of drug treatment: two for allergy to penicillin, one because of gastro-intestinal bleeding caused by aspirin, one for excessive dosage with digitalis and one for an anaemia caused by salazopyrin used in the treatment of ulcerative colitis. In addition there was one addict to pethidine and five cases of drug overdosage taken in a suicidal attempt.

But it is not only drugs that have risks. Surgery, too, and many kinds of investigation, blood transfusion and anaesthesia can go wrong and death may follow. Each year the Registrar General lists the number of deaths in England and Wales from the effects of investigation and treatment. In 1965, excluding accidental overdosage, there were 333: of these 235 followed an adverse drug reaction and 98 were caused by errors of technique.[2]

The Effect on Medicine

Scientific invention and the new drugs have raised the stakes. Supported by a number of highly effective but potentially lethal new drugs, medicine has moved into a new era. Aided by a battery of tests and investigations diagnosis is less the central problem that it was and it can be more accurate, detailed and certain than it used to be. The focus of medicine has moved from diagnosis to therapeutics and other techniques of treatment, and medicine is able to deploy an array of weapons such as it has never had before.

But skill, knowledge and judgment are now more necessary to the doctor than before, when diagnosis was the main aim and the course of the illness for better or for worse had largely to be left to nature. For the patient, with the new drugs and their capacity to do much good and great harm, the risks have been increased. For the doctor the maxim *primum non nocere* has become more difficult to live up to.

Once a diagnosis has been made the doctor's role becomes complex. He knows on the one hand the likely outcome of the illness if it is left untreated, its severity, its unpleasantness, its possibly lasting effects and its complications, and he is under pressure, often informed pressure, from the patient and his relations to act. He knows, too,

[1] Barr, D. P. (1955), *J. Amer. med. Ass.*, **159**, 1452.
[2] *Registrar General's Statistical Review for 1967*. (H.M.S.O. London).

the range of effective remedies available. On the other hand he knows, or should know, their respective merits and their differing liabilities to produce serious side-effects, toxic and allergic reactions. He has to balance these three variables in the equation in his head— seriousness of disease, effectiveness of remedy, liability to side-effects —and to produce an answer.

He has to avoid using a sledgehammer to crack a nut like pre-scribing tetracycline for a pustule, and to refuse to use potent and possibly dangerous drugs like antibiotics for conditions such as a feverish chill in which they are unlikely to help. Equally, he should not hesitate to use effective drugs, even though the risk may be appreciable, if the condition is serious and no other drug is as effective—chloramphenicol, for example, in typhoid fever and streptomycin, often, in pulmonary tuberculosis. If he decides to use a drug despite its hazards he must not use it half-heartedly and run risks but reap little benefit. If he decides, too, to use drugs that are heavy with physiological side-effects such as imipramine for a depressive psychosis, or ganglion-blocking drugs in hypertension, he must explain them to the patient and support him in bearing with them. Lastly, he must resist pressure, from the patient to be given some unsuitable drug, from drug firm representatives to try some new product uncritically, or from inside himself to indulge in what amounts to experiment on human beings, which if he avoids disaster may bring credit and a warm glow to his self-esteem.

It is not surprising, therefore, that the ordinary practitioner has the greatest difficulty in keeping up, in knowing about new drugs, their advantages and drawbacks, in gaining experience in their use and confidence in dealing with their side-effects. In spite of wide reading, of keen attendance at meetings and refresher courses, and of opportunities to talk to specialists at consultations over patients, the keenest practitioner must fall behind, at least in some fields. The plight of the elderly doctor, for whom all the developments in thera-peutics since insulin have happened since he finished training, is worse still.

Because of this, and because chemical and other investigations are available in a hospital, more and more treatment is remaining in the hands of the specialist in his out-patient clinic there. The patient is established on a regime of drug therapy and seen regularly in the clinic for several weeks before returning to the care of his own doctor, or quite commonly, in the case of certain diseases, he may attend a specialised clinic for months or years. Many hospitals have established clinics for the long-term out-patient care of diabetics, hypertensives, for those having corticosteroid drugs or anticoagulant drugs, or for psychiatric patients who are having antidepressant and anti-schizophrenic drug regimes.

This trend, however natural and necessary it may be, has removed much of the interest and excitement from the role of the ordinary doctor, who finds himself on the sidelines, and it has contributed to the present malaise of general practice for which as yet no complete cure has been found.

Besides the devaluation of general practice, specialisation and the shift of medicine's centre of gravity to the hospital have had other effects.

First, the referral system that is so characteristic of British medicine has come under severe strain. The complexity of drug treatment and the necessity for multiple investigations have meant that in referring a patient for a specialist opinion the general practitioner has lost effective control of the patient for weeks or months at a time. Direct access for the general practitioner to hospital laboratories and X-ray departments is a growing facility, but its extension to more sophisticated forms of investigation would serve the dual purpose of helping to prevent the further decay of general practice as a rewarding kind of doctoring and of diminishing the overload on hospital out-patient departments.

If the general practitioner does lose control, who becomes the patient's new anchor? Who is able to see the patient as a person with emotions, problems, a home and family, and not just as a piece of machinery whose physico-chemical systems have gone awry? Ideally the hospital physician or surgeon to whom the patient is originally referred, even if he works in a narrow field, should do this —and many do. But if some specialist is not prepared to act in this role the patient is adrift. There is no one to explain to him what is happening, why further investigations and opinions are necessary, and he is in danger of moving aimlessly from one department to another; as often as not if no abnormality is found the patient is ultimately referred to the psychiatric department for no positive reason. The psychiatrist is faced with a disgruntled patient who has no idea why he is sent and has often no wish to be seen. No one has bothered either to obtain background information or to ask for the general practitioner's views.

This is British hospital doctoring at its worst. But luckily it seldom happens, and it probably happens today less often than it did before the war. Then the dependants of insured people and the uninsured poor often had no doctor of their own, or could not afford a visit.

They were wholly dependent for their medical care on the casualty and out-patient departments of local hospitals with their frequently changing staff; no one knew them over the years save the department's sister. Today, in Britain at least, everyone has the right to his own doctor.

In the past, then, it was the poor and particularly the elderly woman who was in danger of getting lost in the meshes of the hospital system. She could well have no single doctor who knew her and her background and maladies. Today the danger affects a different group of people and has reappeared in a different form. We all revere the expert, which in medicine means the specialist and his retinue of scientific aids. The general practitioner finds it very difficult to resist a patient's demand for specialist advice even if he thinks that it is unnecessary. Some patients, and they tend to be the well informed, virtually refer themselves and in some specialties the consultant acquiesces. As a matter of courtesy the practitioner may be kept informed, but the initiative comes from the patient, who may not be on the right track and may have chosen the wrong department. In some fields, gynaecology and psychiatry perhaps, the patient may not want to disclose personal problems to her or his own doctor and there is a case for self-referral, just as there has always been with venereal disease clinics. This trend towards self-referral, barely discernible in Britain yet, though it is quite clear in the cities of the United States, could become important and dangerous.

Secondly, science and specialised medicine have had an overwhelmingly mechanistic bias. The patient increasingly tends to be regarded as a mass of disordered systems, his human characteristics lost sight of. There is nothing fundamentally untenable, of course, in a mechanist-determinist-behaviourist philosophy as a theoretical model. But behavioural science, though it is developing fast, will have to achieve much more before medicine can adopt this model in the doctor's ordinary task of trying to deal with patients. To equate disease solely with demonstrable physical, chemical and electrical abnormalities is, in the present state of science, naïve. Yet some branches attempt to do so.

Lastly, specialisation has gone so far that the profession is in danger of fragmentation. In surgery, a man may become famous for one particular orthopaedic operation, or for operating only on the thyroid gland or for exclusively repairing arteries. In medicine some superspecialties have developed a language so much their own that communication with the body of medicine is hard to maintain. Immunology, radiotherapy, haematology, and psycho-pharmacology are examples of fields where this is happening and where the ordinary doctor can have the greatest difficulty in understanding the new advances.

This is not to decry the virtues of specialisation, or to argue that a patient is worse off if he is operated on by a surgeon who has perfected a particular technique. No doctor should deliberately undertake any operation for which he has not been properly trained, and attempts to revive or sustain general practice by enabling its practitioners to be jacks-of-all-specialties are badly misguided. They must be master of their own sphere; what is needed is for their sphere, which potentially is a wide one, to be redefined. It should not be entirely divorced from the hospital; as we have seen, because of the intensive specialisation of hospital medicine, there is more scope than there used to be for the generalist, who can explain to the patient what is happening to him. And the general practitioner ought to be able to treat his patients in hospital for illnesses which are within his competence. But there is another direction to which he can look in the future if he fears that his present sphere is contracting. Medicine the world over has three great divisions; after hospital medicine, which thanks to science has attracted all the glamour, and general practice itself comes preventive medicine, never a popular subject even with doctors, and hardly a favourite for the mass media, but which has received a new impetus from scientific advance and the hopes and fears of twentieth century society.

CHAPTER FOUR

Preventive Medicine

It is time to move on and outwards from the consulting room and the bedside to the community, the field of preventive medicine. Science— its techniques and its products, its methods and its drugs—has had the same transforming effect here as it has had on medicine for the individual; but whereas in personal medicine scientific discovery has been of unique and overwhelming importance in moulding its new character, in preventive medicine science has been only one of several causes of change.

Three others stand out: great social and economic changes leading, in this century, to increasing wealth and welfare; the foundation of international institutions, the League of Nations and the United Nations, whose roles in fostering international health have been so remarkable; and conceptual changes wholly of this century such as the possibility born of international action of eradicating some diseases from the world, and the idea that diseases can be diagnosed, again on a large scale, before they have produced symptoms.

As a result, preventive medicine has become a growing point in medicine and is no longer so exclusively concerned as it used to be with drab words—hygiene, quarantine, sanitation and standardised death rates—important though they may be.

Thanks to science the methods and techniques of specific preventive medicine and the drugs used in personal therapeutic medicine have come to be regarded as the twin guardians of the public against infectious disease. This view is incomplete to say the least and is only true of the last thirty years or so. It is quite untrue of the first third of the century.

Chart II (p. 72) shows the death rate from tuberculosis and a select list of infections in the United States and in England and Wales throughout the century. In both countries mortality was falling fast before there were either specific preventive methods for any of these illnesses or specific therapy.

In his analysis of the reasons for the improvement in health in

Britain in the last two centuries Professor McKeown[1] says:

"We owe the advance in health mainly, not to what happens when we are ill, but to the fact that we do not so often become ill. And we remain well, not because of specific preventive measures such as vaccination and immunisation, but because we enjoy a higher standard of living and live in a healthier environment."

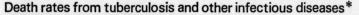 **Death rates from tuberculosis and other infectious diseases*** Chart II

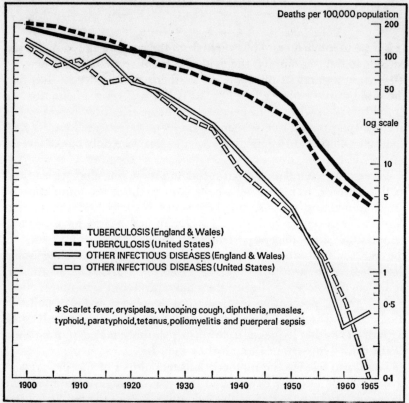

Sources: Vital Statistics of the United States, United States Dept of Health, Education & Welfare, Registrar General's Statistical Reviews.

* Note: 1965 was an epidemic and 1960 an interepidemic year for measles in England and Wales and in 1965 measles caused two thirds of its deaths from "other infectious diseases".

And again:

"Without denying the value of the personal health services, or of the specific therapy which has been a notable achievement of the past

[1] McKeown, T. *Medicine in Modern Society*, pp. 9, 55. (George Allen and Unwin. London, 1965).

forty years, it seems right to conclude that in order of relative importance the main influences responsible for the decline of mortality . . .
have been: a rising standard of living; the control of the physical
environment; and specific preventive and curative therapy."

In the latter half of the nineteenth century improvements in health
resulted from the decrease in poverty, malnutrition, ignorance and
overcrowding as much as from the more specifically medical measures
of sanitary reform. In this century social and economic betterment
has certainly been maintained, with benefit to the nation's health;
in addition, changes peculiar to the century—measures to prevent
poverty broadly summarised as social security, together with town
planning, housing subsidies, subsidised meals and milk for schoolchildren, and numerous services for the elderly—must have paid a
handsome dividend in improved health.

The cost of this social infrastructure is immense and, coupled with
the cost of preventive and personal health services, is a heavy burden
for even the richest countries. For underdeveloped and developing
countries it is prohibitive. Aid for this purpose from richer to poorer
is a drop in the ocean.

International Developments

Infectious disease is international. It is enlightened self-interest, as
well as humanity, that stimulates aid programmes to bring it under
control. Infectious diseases know nothing of national boundaries;
the existence of a pool of infection in one country is a constant threat
to that country's neighbours, and, in these days of speedy travel, to
countries far and wide. In 1963 there were 218 cases of rabies in the
Philippines, and 1,597 cases of diphtheria in Egypt; in 1964 17,000
people died of cholera in India and 513 cases of plague were reported
in Tanzania; in 1964 India had 32,000 cases of smallpox with 9,100
deaths.[1] So long as these reservoirs of serious infection persist, no
advanced country that has managed to control these diseases can
relax.

International measures to control infectious disease are a natural
corollary and by and large they have been a twentieth century
development. The century opened with Gorgas's eradication of
yellow fever from Havana and later from Panama by his attack on
the *Aëdes aegypti* mosquito and its larvae—a tremendous achievement.
At about the same time the Pan-American Sanitary Bureau was

[1] WHO *Epidemiology and Vital Statistics Report* for 1965. (Geneva).

established as an agency of the twenty-one American republics. The opening of this bureau in Washington in 1902 was an event of considerable importance, as it seems to have been the first occasion on which sovereign states yielded some of their sovereignty to an international body; each government pledged itself to aid the bureau in investigating outbreaks of infectious disease within its borders and to allow the bureau to enforce sanitary measures at seaports.[1] It now serves as the regional office in the Western hemisphere of the World Health Organisation.

International co-operation elsewhere followed on the inauguration of the League of Nations and the foundation of its health organisation. The World Health Organisation, an agency of the United Nations, dates from 1948 when it took over the work of the League's health organisation and the health division of UNRRA. Its achievements in so short a time have been massive, not least in the publication of regular reports, bulletins and a wealth of statistical material—too much, indeed, even to summarise here. Instead, it would be better to deal in more detail with one of its most important and successful activities—the control of malaria.

This ancient disease, caused by a microscopic parasite, was, under the name of the ague, not uncommon in England—in the Fen-country, in Essex, and in Kent—until the mid-nineteenth century. Three types of parasite are known, which spend part of their life cycle in man and the remainder in one of 60 varieties of mosquito. Malaria is the world's greatest single cause of disablement. In 1955, 1,100 million of the world's population were exposed to it, 200 million suffered from it, and 2 million people died from it. In the words of a WHO publication,[2] "it stunts physical and mental development, hampers the exploitation of natural resources, reduces agricultural production and impairs industry and commerce." It has been said that in Africa 10–15% of children under four years of age die directly from the disease. It periodically incapacitates its victims and stops them from working, but even in the intervals between acute attacks the sufferers are lethargic, apathetic and work at half capacity.

The disease can be prevented by interfering with the life-cycle of the parasite at any of a number of points: by suppressing the disease in man so that any mosquito which bites him remains uninfected; by abolishing the mosquito's breeding places; by attacking and

[1] Russell, P. F. *Man's Mastery of Malaria.* (Geoffrey Cumberlege: Oxford University Press. London, 1955).
[2] WHO *Malaria Eradication—a plea for health.* (Geneva, 1958).

destroying the larvae; by protecting man from being bitten by means of nets and insect repellents; and by attacking the adult mosquito.

Before the last twenty years it was often possible to control the disease and much reduce its incidence by a considerable effort expended over a small area. Measures like the eradication of stagnant water, the spreading of oil on expanses of still water, prophylactic doses of quinine taken regularly, and the provision of sleeping nets could and did protect people where, as with the armed forces, the sanitary services were well developed and compulsion could be exerted. For example, Gorgas's methods during the building of the Panama canal reduced the yearly rate of admission of the canal workers to hospital for malaria from 821 to 76 per 1,000 in eight years.[1] Prophylaxis by medication of whole populations has been less successful. The extent of the disease can be reduced by this measure, but it cannot be eradicated and, of course, all antimalarial drugs have side-effects.

There is, too, an ever present risk that malarial parasites will develop resistance to all antimalarial drugs. There are already reports that in Thailand[2] and elsewhere one variety of malarial parasite has developed resistance to chloroquine, the most successful antimalarial drug. No doubt, in some cases apparent drug resistance merely conceals the fact that people have not been taking the drug prophylactically either regularly or in sufficient amounts. But American troops in Vietnam have developed malaria while taking prophylactic drugs regularly, and there can be little doubt that resistant strains are multiplying. These reports come not only from the Far East but also from West Africa and South America. In some cases parasites have apparently become resistant to other synthetic antimalarial drugs besides chloroquine at the same time: mepacrine, proguanil and pyrimethamine. Quinine is coming into its own again.

Besides the synthesis of new antimalarial drugs much more effective than quinine, the vastly improved control over malaria during the last twenty years can be attributed to the large-scale production of a range of persistent insecticides and to the organisation on an international scale of teams of specialists to visit malarial areas and to inaugurate control programmes there.

[1] Russell, P. F., op. cit.

[2] "Previously the drug of choice, chloroquine given alone now fails to cure many [malarial] infections in Thailand." Harinasuta, T., Viravan, C. and Reid, A. A. (1967), *Lancet*, **i**, 1117. In the same article these authors describe high success in radically curing resistant cases by combining either chloroquine or pyrimethamine with a single dose of sulphormethoxine, a long-acting sulphonamide drug.

Without disparaging the importance of other measures—drainage, spraying of breeding places and so forth—there are firm grounds for saying that the greatest single advance has been the regular spraying of the insides of all dwellings in the area under attack with residual insecticide (either D.D.T. Gammexane, Dieldrin or Chlordane).

As a consequence of the success of local efforts to control malaria the new concept of eradication has become a practical proposition. As long ago as 1945 Venezuela announced a plan to eradicate the disease from the entire country. Residual spraying twice a year was the main weapon. Since then many other countries have announced similar programmes and some have achieved their goal. The eighth World Health Assembly in 1955 set eradication rather than control as the aim. The complete elimination of the disease from the world is now not an impossible prospect.

The first and essential step is a political one. An afflicted country has to decide that it will devote funds and resources to the end of malaria eradication. Technical aid and money are then available from international sources. On request WHO will send a demonstration team to study local conditions—the local species of mosquito, its sensitivity to insecticides, its habits, the wall surface of local buildings and the best methods of spraying. The team helps in the recruitment of staff, in training them, and in giving demonstrations of spraying techniques. All this may take a year. The attack phase follows. Every dwelling is sprayed twice or more a year for three or four years.

Once transmission of the disease from mosquito to man and *vice versa* has been stopped for this span of time there will be no parasites left in man or mosquito. Spraying can be stopped and the country enters what has been called the phase of consolidation. All remaining reservoirs of human infection have to be sought out and energetically treated. It is customary now to regard malaria as eliminated if during another three years of surveillance no new cases are found.

The final phase is one of maintenance. Measures have to be taken against reintroduction of the disease from abroad, and each fresh case which does appear has to be promptly investigated and treated, in particular to ensure that the patient does not infect any mosquito that happens to bite him.

By 1966 the Director General of WHO was able to report[1] that very large parts of the Americas and South-East Asia and the whole of continental Europe were free of endemic malaria. Programmes covering a population of 626 million people were progressing well

[1] WHO. *Annual Report of Director General.* (Geneva, 1966).

within the planned time-limit. In India areas with over half the population of the originally malarious regions are now in the maintenance phase. But in places there have been delays and setbacks, and in Tobago after a malaria-free interval of thirteen years the disease had a short-lived resurgence.

The cost of these eradication programmes *in toto* is large, but when measured against human suffering averted is tiny. It varies from about 15 U.S. cents for each person protected in South-East Asia to 50 cents in the Western hemisphere. Before it was fully understood that the attack need only be pursued for a limited number of years and that spraying need not be continued indefinitely the mounting and continuing cost of these eradication projects was alarming. Now that it is known that the link in the chain need only be broken for four years or so poor countries are much reassured and encouraged to pursue their programmes vigorously in the interest of economy as well as of health.

The total eradication of the insect vector would be much more expensive and difficult to achieve. Indeed it might be impossible. By 1958 there were reports that four out of sixty known insect vectors had developed resistance to commonly used insecticides. This phenomenon does not imply that any individual insect develops resistance to drugs during its lifetime. The sensitive insect remains sensitive and is killed before it can multiply, whereas inherently resistant strains continue to multiply regardless of a concentration of insecticide many times that which would suffice to destroy its sensitive fellows. Resistant strains of mosquito have given trouble in Panama, in Greece and in Java, but the difficulties have been overcome. Nevertheless there is an urgency about the eradication programme. Even if strains of mosquito resistant to insecticides have so far failed to upset it, the worse threat, the spread of strains of malarial parasite resistant to antimalarial drugs, remains. There are indeed reports that American servicemen are bringing resistant strains of parasite back to the United States and that these are infecting the local mosquitoes in Texas.[1] We may have an opportunity that will never recur. Perhaps it is already lost. Is malaria slipping in through the front door while people are so preoccupied with pushing it out of the back?

Success in eradicating malaria from vast areas of the world's surface will have far-reaching consequences. Ill-health, lethargy, and inefficiency in formerly affected populations should diminish and the potential benefit to the economies of such countries can hardly be guessed at. Simultaneously, success will hugely intensify the pressure

[1] *Medical News.* 17 March, 1967.

of population growth and make a tolerable solution to this problem more urgently necessary than ever. There should also be some encouragement both to suffering member countries and to international organisations—and to fund-giving foundations—to tackle other widespread diseases. Indeed this is already happening. Yellow fever, another mosquito-borne disease but caused by a virus; bilharziasis, a disease in which the vector is a snail that flourishes in rivers and in irrigation canals; trypanosomiasis, the African disease transmitted by the tsetse fly; ankylostomiasis, caused by the hook-worm; these and many more are examples of widespread disease in which money and men for field study and research, modern insecticides, molluscicides and other drugs could transform life for the afflicted populations.

Migration

In the case of infectious diseases that travel, like malaria, yellow fever, smallpox, diphtheria, plague and tuberculosis the humanitarian impulses of the developed countries that contribute most to the resources of international control bodies are reinforced by a strong element of self-interest. The steep rise in air travel carries the constant risk of infected people being transported to distant countries during the incubation period of a disease, and of insect vectors of some diseases travelling too. There is a danger of epidemics, of which public health doctors are only too well aware. An attack on disease in its endemic strongholds would entail a vast international effort; it would be only likely to succeed if it were coupled with even more vast economic and social improvements—better nutrition, less poverty and overcrowding—changes which, to say the least, are going to take some time to achieve. Nevertheless the announcement that WHO included a sum of $2·4 million in its budget for 1966 to make a start on eradicating endemic smallpox is very welcome indeed.

Public health problems have been created too by the tides of immigration, which in their present form are a postwar phenomenon. The immense shifts of population entailed by great wars have always produced risks of widespread epidemics, of course, but in peacetime in this century (apart from pilgrimages to Mecca) the migrations of population have until lately mainly been from areas where standards of hygiene and public health were high. The chief exception—emigration to the United States—has for a long time been complicated by the demand of the health authorities there for a medical examination before entry. Now that Britain has accepted large-scale immigration from the Indian subcontinent, from Africa, and the West Indies the risks to health have aroused some concern, and the need for some kind of examination before entry is generally accepted.

Most concern has been over tuberculosis. In cities like Bradford, with a sizeable Asian immigrant population, more than half of the new cases of tuberculosis are found to occur in immigrants, especially in those from Pakistan,[1] and the incidence in them may well be thirty times that in the British population.[2] Another study[3] has found the notification-rate to be for Indians twelve times and for Pakistanis twenty-six times that of the indigenous population. Possibly more than half of these patients have developed the disease since their arrival. Certainly such factors as low innate resistance, an unfamiliar and much more severe climate, and overcrowding would encourage its spread, but these would be of much less importance were it not for the prevalence of unsuspected infectious cases. No one knows accurately how many immigrants have the disease when they come, but it seems likely that 20–40% of the cases coming to light may fall into this category. And they more often than not harbour drug-resistant strains, possibly because of self-medication with preparations containing anti-tuberculous drugs in inadequate doses.

The importation and local spread of a disease that has only lately been brought under control is disquieting. The remedy is not easy to find. It is said that 10–20 million people die of tuberculosis each year. Control of the disease in Asia is remote. India alone is thought to have six million cases, a quarter of them infectious. By 1965, 80 million had had vaccination with BCG, but this vast preventive effort has barely kept pace with the increase in the population over the same period of fifteen years.[4]

Until 1968 British Government policy was against a compulsory examination of intending immigrants in their home countries; facilities are, in any case, so scanty that such examination may be incomplete or unreliable. Control after entry, despite the best efforts at case finding on the part of the local authorities mainly at risk, has proved disappointing. In Bradford advertising, canvassing and lectures have not been successful in inducing the immigrants to come for X-rays, and it seems very doubtful whether the advice of the Government to the immigrant to get himself on the list of a doctor, and to the doctor to consider the need for a chest X-ray, is any more

[1] *Lancet*, (1965), **i**, 150.
[2] Stevenson, D. K. (1962), *Brit. Med. J.*, **i**, 1382.
[3] Thomas, H. E. (1968), *Proc. Roy. Soc. Med.*, **61**, 21.
[4] O'Rourke, J. O. (1965), *Lancet*, **ii**, 128.

likely to be followed. An X-ray at his place of work has more chance of success than any other method once the immigrant has left the port of entry. Most health authorities, however, consider that despite the political and administrative difficulties some kind of compulsion is justifiable on immigrants from high-risk areas—either an X-ray before or on entry[1] or compulsory attendance at a local chest clinic soon afterwards—to avert the threat of the introduction into the country of strains resistant to several of the commonly used anti-tuberculous drugs and their spread to fellow-Asians and ultimately perhaps to the indigenous population.

For the moment tuberculosis is the main hazard of the postwar wave of immigration. There is much less concern about the possible introduction of tropical diseases or of other diseases like smallpox, diphtheria and typhoid, for decades of experience of prevention have yielded good control which is unlikely to break down. But immigrants, like armies, have always had a higher incidence of venereal disease than the native population. This is a fact of the epidemiology of syphilis and gonorrhoea and is as true of Puerto Ricans in New York as of West Indians in Britain. In part it is related to the stress of life in an alien culture, in part to the type of person who emigrates. The men usually come first without their wives or possible wives and for a time lead a socially isolated lodging-house life. Venereal disease in a narrow sense is a public health problem, but more broadly it is, for these reasons, a social problem akin to alcoholism and to drug addiction, and likely to remain one until either the immigrant has been accepted in his new society or until he and his compatriots have built their new community within the host society. It follows that social policy—obstacles that stop them from obtaining housing and delay in enabling wives to join husbands—directly influences the health of immigrants and hosts alike.[2]

Screening (*Presymptomatic Diagnosis*)

In a sense the compulsory examination of immigrants on entry to a country is a variety of screening, but this is to use the word in an antique sense. In a sense, too, anyone who enters the armed forces or who undergoes an examination for life insurance is screened, or, in

[1] Over 9,000 X-rays of immigrants on entry at London Airport, 1965–66, disclosed 85 positive cases (9·2 per 1,000). Kinsella, F. J. G. (1968), *Proc. Roy. Soc. Med.*, **61**, 23.

[2] In England and Wales in 1965 half the cases in men of gonorrhoea and 40% of the new male cases of early infectious syphilis were in immigrants. Dolton, W. D. (1968), *Proc. Roy. Soc. Med.*, **61**, 19. These percentages have been roughly confirmed for 1967 by the Chief Medical Officer of the Ministry of Health.

modern parlance, has a "health check". Such examinations are time-consuming and expensive and also highly unreliable, certainly when carried out by a doctor in haste because he has a large number of examinations to perform. It is a boring procedure for the doctor, and people have been known to slip through unnoticed when they have such gross abnormalities as a heart on the right side of their chests. But "screening" in its accepted sense of performing a single test or examination of a limited area or function is of much more value. It began as a result of the technical advance that enabled mass miniature radiography to be done during the war, and in 1966 as many as 3·26 million mass radiography examinations were made in England and Wales. It is difficult to say whether this, because it identifies the early case, has done more than the development of antituberculous drugs, the BCG vaccination or a higher standard of living in reducing the number of deaths from pulmonary tuberculosis in people under thirty from 6,000 to 18 a year in the last twenty-two years.

Tuberculosis is an infectious disease, but the more recent developments in "screening" have been designed to discover other conditions, particularly cancer. If one asks why miniature radiography should not be used to detect lung cancer in its early stages the answer is that by the time the growth is visible on an X-ray film it is often too late to operate with much hope of success. A better hope in this disease is to examine specimens of sputum to find cancer cells. This might be an examination to which heavy smokers should submit themselves at intervals. But results, so far, are disappointing.

At present various kinds of screening are undertaken in Britain, notably the routine testing of babies' urine for phenylpyruvic acid. This is done by a simple impregnated paper test. A positive result indicates that the child suffers from phenylketonuria, a genetic disease affecting about one in twelve thousand children. It is caused by a recessive gene, and as a consequence the child develops mental defect unless it is fed from an early age on a diet free from the amino-acid phenylalanine.[1]

Cancer of the cervix of the uterus caused 2,449 deaths in England and Wales in 1967. Twenty-five years ago Papanicolaou and Traut published a monograph[2] on the detection of uterine cancer by a cervical smear. It is claimed that in trained hands this enables a diagnosis of early cancer to be made and also detects precancerous

[1] The screening test has come in for criticism lately. It is too insensitive. A more complex urine test or a blood test is more efficient. (*Brit. Med. J.*, 1968, **4,** 7).
[2] Papanicolaou, G. N. and Traut, H. F. *Diagnosis of Uterine Cancer by Vaginal Smear*. Commonwealth Fund. (New York, 1943).

F

conditions of the cervix. If precancerous conditions or very early malignancies are picked out in this way the outlook with surgery is very good indeed. This is, unfortunately, a test in which great experience is needed for the result to be reliable, and otherwise experienced pathologists, who have a great deal of other work to do, would probably regard themselves as less reliable in their reports than a trained technician who is doing this work all the time. The trend has therefore been towards specialised clinics entirely devoted to this work and to training qualified technicians solely for it.

In June 1967, 119,000 women in the age group mainly at risk were being screened each month in England and Wales; 605 technicians trained in cytology were at work and others were being trained. That the cost is considerable can be judged from the fact that because the work is exacting and tiring a technician can do only 30 examinations a day.

Less has been heard of screening for cancer of the breast, although in a project in British Columbia it has been carried out to the extent of 100,000 women a year since 1949. This form of cancer causes about a quarter of the deaths from cancer in women, and since with present methods of treatment, surgery and radiotherapy, mortality is not decreasing, emphasis is being placed on early diagnosis. Various methods of screening have been employed, regular self-examination, routine regular examination of the breast by doctors, and the use of soft-tissue radiography (mammography). Unfortunately all the methods used so far consume a prohibitive amount of doctor-time and attention is now turning to the identification of a high-risk group which could then be regularly and systematically examined. This group would contain those without children, particularly if they have a family history of the disease, and those who have a high level of steroid excretion.

Screening techniques are being evolved for malignant cells in the urine of those exposed to the industrial risk of bladder cancer. Workers in the dyestuffs and the rubber industries are exposed to this hazard.

Glaucoma, an eye disease associated with an insidious rise in tension inside the eye, is responsible for the blindness of one in seven of the registered blind; it causes 800 new cases of blindness each year; and 40% of those who go blind from glaucoma have not been diagnosed and treated for the condition until they have become blind, for symptoms can be very late in appearing. Early detection, therefore, is sight-saving and screening of whole populations, particularly of the age chiefly at risk, has been done in the United States for some time and has recently been introduced in Britain. In a clinic devoted to this purpose in Bedford[1] the first 2,000 cases screened yielded 1·6% of people who had definite glaucoma—people presumably in whom a diagnosis would otherwise not have been made for some time. This figure is about the same as has been found in similar surveys in the United States. Of the total number screened about 8% have to be referred for further investigation and assessment. The test consists of asking about the family history, asking if the patient has had attacks of blurred vision or seen haloes round naked lights at night, and then the use of a tonometer to measure the intraocular tension.

The whole concept of screening for this disease has not escaped criticism. The criteria for an established diagnosis and the screening methods are by no means universally agreed, and some doctors fear that because one variety of glaucoma can be intermittent a number of people with glaucoma will be missed in any survey. Another group in whom the findings are on the borderline will be subjected, perhaps needlessly, to repeated examinations over a period of years and to much harmful anxiety about their eyes. As with high blood pressure the significance of raised intraocular tension is not entirely clear. Some people, found at screening to have raised tension, have been watched for some years and many have not developed glaucoma. On the other hand, the field defects of glaucoma can develop at quite low pressure. In spite of these criticisms, which could equally well be made of screening for pulmonary tuberculosis, the discovery of 16 cases per 1,000 of population screened is probably very worth while.

Screening techniques could suitably apply, if it is possible to develop them, to any diseases with the following characteristics: the disease should not be rare, or, if it is, early discovery should be absolutely essential for effective treatment as it is in phenylketonuria; it should not be trivial; it should be silent in its early stages and amenable to treatment when discovered; there should be widespread agreement on diagnostic criteria; the test should be simple, painless and highly discriminating with a very low proportion of doubtful, false positive, and false negative results.

Screening of populations of apparently normal people for diabetes has been carried out sporadically for at least ten years. The procedure used to have two stages: the identification by a simple impregnated paper test of those who pass sugar in their urine after a main meal; further tests, including blood tests, on this select group, for only a small percentage—about a quarter—of these turn out to have overt

[1] Perkins, E. S. (1965), *Brit. Med. J.*, **i,** 417

diabetes. Recently, blood tests have been exclusively used in screening. About five people in a thousand in any community are known diabetics. Reports on screening tests have shown that a further five people have diabetes without knowing it. These need treatment. Another four people have abnormalities of a minor sort, but their importance is unclear at present. Are the ranks of future diabetics recruited from them or not? Should they be kept under regular observation or should attention be concentrated, as has been suggested,[1] on those people known to have a much higher risk of developing the disease than others—relatives of known diabetics, the obese, and people over 50?

In the United States screening has gone much further than this. People with no symptoms have undergone routine tests at mass examinations by "multiple screening", not only tests for sugar in the urine, for glaucoma and for tuberculosis and syphilis. They have also had a urine test for albumen, had their blood pressure measured and an electrocardiogram taken, and in some surveys blood counts and sight testing. Such examinations reveal of course occasional cases of serious disease and abnormality that need attention. More often they show a much larger number of people to have a minor abnormality, perhaps a mildly raised blood pressure or some slightly unusual pattern in the electrocardiogram, the exact significance of which is unknown. We know far too little of the natural history of diseases of the heart and blood vessels to be able to say whether incidental findings like these in people with no symptoms carry any threat, whether "treatment" has any effect, or even whether the patient's own knowledge of the abnormal finding may not in itself be harmful.

Blunderbuss screening of the general health check kind not only reveals a proportion of people with abnormalities that are difficult to evaluate. It may also fail to reveal a disease that is lethal. An American report[2] from ten clinics engaged in making periodic examinations of people actively engaged in industry and university work discloses some of the inadequacies of this kind of routine examination. The tests were thorough and included a complete history of the patient and a complete physical examination; examination of the urine and faeces, of the lower bowel through a sigmoidoscope, of the blood for sedimentation rate, anaemia, cholesterol and sugar; electrocardiogram and chest X-ray. The authors were especially interested in 350 people who had died at some time after

[1] Crombie, D. I. (1962), *Proc. Roy. Soc. Med.*, **55**, 205.
[2] Schor, S. S., Clark, T. W., Parkhurst, L. W., Baber, J. P. and Elsom, K. A. (1964), *Ann. int. Med.*, **61**, 999.

one or more of these health checks. Just over half of them died of coronary attacks and a fifth of cancer. The disease that killed them or one closely related to it was recognised at the last examination in only 51% and the existence of disease was recognised much more often in the elderly and in those whose death happened less than six months after an examination. However, 42% of those who died of coronary artery disease and 57% of those who died of cancer did so without their disease being discovered at their last health check. The authors, who were, and still are, enthusiasts for this kind of examination, have shown its limitations, and these should be clearly understood by the public. A negative health check, even if it is recent, does not entitle anyone to ignore symptoms.

It has been suggested[1] that multiple screening may be less suited to conditions in Britain, where the health service enables a patient to visit his doctor as soon as he gets any symptoms, than in America, where the cost of a visit may inhibit him. This argument ignores the existence of a group of people, an unknown proportion, who will attend for screening because they think that they have nothing wrong with them but who, if they have symptoms, delay consulting their doctors because they fear that some serious condition will be found. If early diagnosis and the opportunity of early treatment are the aim, it seems unwise for people to wait for symptoms to drive them to see a doctor. Screening techniques, so long as they are simple, not too costly in terms of the effort needed to identify a single case, reliable, and designed to identify a sizeable group, are clearly here to stay; they need to be refined and applied to groups of the population known to be particularly at risk.

It seems that the towns of Salford and Rotherham and lately the city of Glasgow are the only authorities in Britain so far to offer a health check on the American scale. The local health service in Salford[2] offers tests covering "cancer and lung diseases, blood pressure, vision, diabetes, anaemia and weight". This all takes half-an-hour and abnormalities are reported to the patient's doctor. "Last year, over the two-month period available, [the full range of tests were] taken by nearly 3,500 adults. Thousands of others took part of the tests." The population at risk is 154,000. In Rotherham in 1966 5,763 attended from a population of 87,000. Is this a new pattern of medical care emerging—à l'américaine? The best guess is probably Yes—this is here to stay—with suitable modifications to make the tests more directed, more specific, more able to yield usable

[1] Wilson, J. M. G. (1963), Lancet, ii, 51.
[2] Observer, 17 January, 1965.

information. After all, that old emblem of the doctor, the stethoscope, has changed its function. It is still used in estimating the blood pressure, but as an instrument for giving useful information in chest diseases it has, except for the punctilious, been all but superseded by the chest X-ray. Just as this in its screening guise has discovered new patients who did not know that they should be patients, refined screening techniques may yield material for preventive medicine. To be for the moment a trifle fantastic, it is not impossible that a routine analysis of the serum-immunoglobulins might predict those liable to develop ulcerative colitis, or that screening of the relatives of schizophrenics for the level of 5-hydroxytryptamine and 3, 4-dimethoxyphenylethylamine in the blood might identify those likely to become schizophrenic too.

But any pronounced trend towards regular health checks of these specific kinds will need a change in outlook on the public's part and a change in orientation on the part of doctors. The public will have to be educated to understand just what can and what cannot be discovered by these routine checks and doctors to regard attendance as prudent rather than unhealthily hypochondriacal. This should not be too difficult to bring about, for the same attitude to preventive dentistry is already accepted. It is impractical to expect general practitioners in present circumstances actually to carry out health check procedures—these would have to be specially organised within the public health programme—but a change in attitude would be necessary. A degree of concentration on early diagnosis, surveillance of those shown by screening to have borderline abnormalities, encouragement of high-risk groups of people to attend for screening —these and other measures should not be too difficult, too positive, or too time-consuming for general practitioners to take in the interests of prevention—in fact the despised general practitioner may here find a new and invaluable role. Some radical changes will be necessary in medical education, where the full-blown classical case still holds the centre of the clinical stage and the student's interest.

Screening is indeed a new field for the preventive medicine experts of advanced countries now that infectious diseases have been so largely contained. Elsewhere these experts are still fully occupied in fighting infectious diseases with more or less success.

Present Problems

The combination of steeply falling death-rates from infectious disease and preventive medicine's new preoccupation with screening for non-infectious disease could easily give rise to the impression that infection has been defeated. For many reasons this impression is premature.

It is true that successes are still being chalked up—the control of poliomyelitis being the most recent. Now it seems that measles is being brought under control with a live attenuated vaccine. In the United States four years' experience with large-scale use of this vaccine has reduced the number of cases to the lowest on record.[1] Trials have been going on in Britain, too, for three years with encouraging results and a report from Oxford[2] shows that the number of cases notified in 1967, an epidemic year, was even below the number in recent inter-epidemic years. In consequence, the Ministry of Health in 1968 launched a nationwide programme of measles vaccination It is true, too, that a breakthrough in the treatment (rather than prevention) of viral diseases may be imminent.

But old enemies still show fight and the increase in many countries of cases of gonorrhoea[3] and the less common syphilis is causing alarm. The phenomenon is worldwide and social factors and some more exlusively medical ones are involved. According to a WHO publication[4] early syphilis has shown a steady rise in 76 countries from the trough it reached in 1955, so that in many of them the number of new cases has reached the high levels recorded at the end of the war. Apart from social causes a main medical reason seems to be that though originally both the gonococcus and the spirochaete of syphilis were sensitive to penicillin the former soon acquired resistance to it. The spirochaete still remains sensitive, but penicillin is now much less often used in the treatment of gonorrhoea and, indeed, because allergy to penicillin is a recognised risk, it is less often used for trivial reasons or even for other serious infections. The tetracycline antibiotics, which today are more commonly used, are rather ineffective against syphilis. Many people, therefore, whose latent or early syphilitic infection was formerly cured by penicillin given for gonorrhoea, or for some other infection, now develop the disease.

This is just one curious example of the surprises that medicine has had to contend with in recent years in the age-old struggle between man and infecting organisms. There are many others and no doubt there will be many more. Unexpectedness is the thread that links

[1] National Communicable Diseases Centre. *Morbidity and Mortality.* (1967), 16. No. 40 333.
[2] Warin, J. F. (1968), *Lancet*, **i,** 410.
[3] In the United States cases of gonorrhoea increased by 24% between 1963 and 1966.
[4] WHO. *Chronicle.* (1964). **18,** 451.

the following instances; in mentioning them it is difficult to avoid endowing these minute enemies with anthropomorphic imputations of wiliness. Satisfactory scientific explanations have been found for all of them, but this does not make it any easier to predict what new tricks these organisms will get up to next.

In the first flush of enthusiasm for penicillin the staphylococcus was among those organisms found to be sensitive. Some years later resistant strains began to give trouble in individual illnesses and then to produce outbreaks of cross-infection in hospital wards. Patients admitted for some simple surgical operation have died from a staphylococcal infection acquired in hospital.

More recently it has been shown that resistance to drugs can be transferred from one species of organism to another by contact in the intestine. Such resistance can be multiple and can make many antibiotics useless in the treatment of severe intestinal infections. Pathologists suspect that this transferable resistance comes from the misuse of antibiotics in treating trivial human infections and perhaps from misuse in promoting growth, rather than in treating disease, in animals.

Soon after the tetracycline broad-spectrum antibiotics were introduced occasional cases were reported in which, after a series of treatments with various antibiotics, patients died of "super-infections" with yeast-like organisms. These massive infections were hitherto unknown. All sensitive types of bacteria, both harmless and harmful, in the intestinal tract had been so reduced in numbers that the growth of the yeasts, which are resistant to antibiotics, luxuriated in the absence of any competition.

Poliomyelitis in endemic form has a long history and small epidemics were recorded in the nineteenth century. The first big epidemic was in the United States in 1916 and it caused 6,000 deaths, 2,000 of them in New York City.[1] A striking feature of that and later epidemics was that, whereas poliomyelitis used to be predominantly a disease of children, in these years many adults were seriously infected. It was many years before it was clearly shown that improved hygiene, by protecting children from infection of the intestinal tract with the virus in early childhood, an infection that seldom produces paralysis, left them with no natural resistance to the disease later in life. This seems a cruel reward for good hygiene and sanitary habits.

In 1962 there were fewer cases of whooping cough notified than ever before. In the following two years the numbers increased, and the illness appeared in those who had been protected with the

[1] Wilson, J. R. *Margin of Safety.* (Collins. London, 1963).

vaccine which, until lately, it was thought might in time completely eradicate the disease in Britain. It now appears[1][2] that a new sub-type of organism has emerged, against which the vaccine strains at present employed are less effective. To regain control the public health workers may have to change the composition of the vaccine. In the last three years deaths have again fallen to a very low figure— twenty to thirty each year.

The concept of eradication of a disease has two meanings: the absence of any cases of a disease over a period of years; or the impossibility of any cases arising because the infecting organism has vanished. It is conceivable that eradication in the latter sense on a world scale—and it must of course be global—might be achieved in the case of a few diseases such as malaria where the infecting organism has obligatory hosts. If the link is broken, so that no parasites infect any man or any mosquito, although other varieties of parasite may flourish in birds, the protozoon cannot exist on its own. Bacteria, however, can live for many years outside the human body, and some have spore forms that can exist for decades. Viruses, even more pertinently, can assume crystalline forms, and presumably they are capable, even after centuries, of infecting once they enter a cell. For diseases caused by bacteria and viruses one can only speak of eradication of disease in a limited sense. In the foreseeable future the best hope of eradicating infectious disease is to maintain the general measures of preventive medicine and to pursue active pro-grammes of immunisation against specific diseases. At the present time it is essential to keep as high a proportion as possible of the population immune to poliomyelitis,[3] smallpox and tuberculosis by vaccination and to diphtheria and tetanus by toxoid inoculation. This policy, in the case of smallpox, is hard to sustain when its opponents can claim that more deaths in most years in Britain are caused by vaccination than by the disease itself.[4] The remedy lies in trying to make vaccination safer, and there are reasonable hopes that this can be done. When infectious diseases of these kinds cease to be endemic in large areas of Asia and Africa the time may come for a re-examination of vaccination.

[1] Preston, N. W. (1965), *Brit. Med. J.*, **ii,** 11.
[2] Wilson, A. T., Henderson, I. R. Moore, E. J. H. and Heywood, S. N. (1965), *Brit. Med. J.* **ii,** 623.
[3] At present in English towns it is probable that the proportion of three to five years olds immunised against poliomyelitis is not higher than two out of three.
[4] In the ten years 1956–65 there were 29 deaths in England and Wales from smallpox. In the same ten years there were 38 deaths from generalised vaccinia following vaccination and from post-vaccinal encephalitis.

It is always possible that a new virus, or a variant of an old one, will, for reasons we do not know, suddenly cause a pandemic or widespread epidemics. This has happened before with, for example, the virus of influenza and the virus of epidemic encephalitis. In pessimistic but far-sighted manner Burnet[1] has raised the grisly spectre of the "escape" of a laboratory virus groomed in experiments in genetics for high virulence and a serological character different from any known virus so that there would be no natural resistance to its attack. The devastation caused could rival that of the more talked-of thermonuclear catastrophe, and perhaps the safeguards against this happening should be as stringent as human ingenuity can make them. So far, the possibility of such a disaster has hardly been mentioned in public.

Preventive medicine needs to go on being concerned, as before, with infectious disease. It needs to be vigilant both on the domestic scene and, because of migration, internationally. But many of its new facets are not concerned with infectious disease at all. They are bringing preventive medicine back into the whole body of medicine, breaking down barriers and diminishing, in Britain particularly, the tripartite isolation that was built into the National Health Service Act of 1946.

In screening, for example, the public health clinics require help from the general practitioner to find the high-risk group and help from the hospital both in further investigation and in the treatment of "positives". The shortage of hospital beds, too, and the high cost of running them have led to the early discharge of patients, particularly in the case of maternity departments. These patients need after-care services, a local health authority responsibility, to be promptly provided. Liaison must be efficient.

But two other features of the twentieth century scene have done more than anything else to bring practitioners of preventive medicine and their staff back into the mainstream: the increase in the proportion of the population who are elderly, have chronic diseases, and need aid for their welfare as well as treatment for their health; and the developments in psychiatry that have led to an increase in the numbers of mentally disabled people in the community and who need aftercare and preventive services. These two topics will be more fully explored in the following chapters.

[1] Burnet, F. M. (1966), *Lancet*, **i**, 37.

CHAPTER FIVE

Population Problems I: The Growth of Populations

Exploding Populations

In the advanced countries of the West, as we have seen, economic advance, preventive medicine, and therapeutic discovery have joined hands to achieve a steep fall in the mortality of the young. An inevitable consequence has been an ageing population, a population in which a high proportion of people reach old age. This is the outstanding feature of the population profile of these countries.

Elsewhere in the world the chief characteristic is the steep increase in numbers—the population explosion. As this is a strong candidate for the head of the list of the world's worst problems it must be discussed first. To what extent has medicine been responsible and what can medicine do to solve it?

The fall in mortality in the eighteenth and later nineteenth century Britain can be credited mostly to economic betterment and much less to the great sanitary measures of Chadwick and Simon. Therapeutic discovery has only had any effect on mortality much more recently, in our own time. In the past wealth had the greater effect. Today, medicine in its twin forms of scientific discovery and specific preventive medicine bears much more responsibility. In the underdeveloped countries, despite all the emphasis laid on economic development and on the need for wealth and welfare to accompany each other, welfare, in the form of medical science, has come first. Or rather, simply because once the answer to health problems—the way to combat the big killing diseases of these countries—was known, and because in the World Health Organisation a body was there to apply it on an international scale, the knowledge was applied. The fruits of medical progress have ripened before the seed of economic betterment has had time to grow, indeed sometimes before it has been planted. The way to abolish poverty in Africa, Asia and Latin America is less clearly attainable than advance in health.

Earlier in this century a high birth rate in these continents was balanced by a high infant mortality rate. There is therefore, in contrast to the demographic picture of Western nations, no large generation born forty or fifty years ago that has survived and now, thanks to modern medicine, will become grandparents. So the population of underdeveloped countries is young. Although their youth, by comparison with an ageing Britain, would seem to present fewer problems, in fact their youthful populations, because economic advance has not kept pace with medical progress, lack the West's opportunities for employment and so for growing richer. Thus, a larger population of fertile age is retaining the reproductive pattern of an earlier period of high mortality without having the means to rear its offspring.

There seem to be only four ways to avoid mass starvation—which has already been seen in parts of India: wholesale slaughter in war; far more aid to promote economic development than the West has yet given; migration on a large scale; and birth control. The first, one hopes, will be avoided and migration is unlikely because of growing restrictiveness on the part of recipient nations. Aid is being given all too reluctantly. The fourth solution involves medicine and is an example of how, in our country, doctors have become entangled in social issues and in dealing with well people.

Though familiar, the figures of population growth never cease to be alarming: the world population in mid-1965 was estimated to be 3,308 millions; since 1900 it has been increasing by one-third every fifteen years; in Latin America the increase is about 3% a year; every five years India's population increases by more than the total population of Great Britain.

It is said that the world death rate has fallen from 26 per 1,000 before the last war to 16 recently. Clearly the more successful the massive international campaigns to eradicate infectious disease are the more they exacerbate the danger. For example, an intensive campaign to eliminate malaria in Mauritius in 1946–48 was so successful that infant mortality fell from 150 to 50 per 1,000 live births, and the death-rate fell from 28 to 10 per 1,000. The total population rose by 40% in ten years.[1]

The neo-Malthusians, those who scent catastrophe in the population explosion and say that the increase is far outrunning any possible expansion in world food supply, do not have the field to themselves. Mr Colin Clark,[2] for example, believes that, as in the past, popula-

---

[1] Burnet, F. M. (1961). *Eugen. Rev.*, **53**, 25.
[2] Clark, C. *Population Growth and Land Use*. (Macmillan. London, 1967).

tion growth, even on the scale that is happening today, will prove to be such a stimulus to agricultural and economic development that the bogy will be laid. But such optimists are in a small minority. To the majority control of births seems an urgent necessity.

Birth Control

This can take three forms: abortion, which is the most drastic, and the least appropriate to the world population problem—although it certainly played an important part in Japan's successful programme of population control; sterilisation, which for psychological reasons is much more acceptable to women than to men; and contraception, of which the newer methods, the Pill and the IUCD, like abortion and sterilisation very much involve the medical profession. In under-developed countries all these methods have been used in programmes of population control. Elsewhere the demand for birth control, the deliberate limitation of size of family, has sprung from individuals themselves and not from government policy. In fact, official policy in many countries has often been unhelpful, if not so positively hostile as is the Roman Catholic Church.

To aid population control Western countries can contribute resources, technical knowledge and trained people through international agencies, but the countries with teeming populations will themselves have to accept population control as a pre-eminent aim even though it may conflict with their cultural habits and religious beliefs—and they will have to spend money on it. In its second five-year plan India allocated $14 million to malaria control and only $10 million to the control of population. The fourth five-year plan, however, calls for $200 million to be spent on the latter. Sometimes, too, the effect of social legislation, desirable on other grounds, favours expansion rather than control. In Chile, for example, pre-natal bonuses and family allowances have encouraged early marriage and larger families.[1] In furthering population control it might have been preferable, as Dr Cruz-Coke suggests, to pay every woman each month for not having a baby.

The longing of women to be free of the tyranny of repeated pregnancy; the crippling effect of the large size of a family on its standard of living; psychological theories asserting that an unwanted child may be handicapped throughout its life; above all, the knowledge that means are at hand to control what had hitherto been haphazard —these are some of the reasons for the revolt of women and their

[1] Cruz-Coke, R. (1965). *Lancet*, **ii**, 434.

husbands against the entrenched forces of social custom and religious authority. Medicine, from Marie Stopes onwards, has been heavily involved.

The twin techniques of modern contraception and artificial insemination have enabled sexual activity to be completely divorced from reproduction for the first time in human history. So long as they were indissolubly tied together society's concern in the number of the young and the welfare of a growing family had to be accompanied by a restriction of free sexual expression, enforced by society's moral and religious attitudes. Nowadays, thanks in part to the triumphs of preventive and curative medicine, it is no longer necessary for families to contain a large number of children in order to replenish the population. Anything much beyond this one-for-one replacement contains the threat of over-population. Enough children can be guaranteed to issue from a tiny fraction of a people's total sexual activity—and that, being instinctively determined, is hardly capable of much modification even by the most stringent laws or by social disapproval. It is not surprising therefore that the taboos on other forms of sexual activity that are designed not to result in children are weakening. These include protected marital intercourse, protected premarital and extramarital intercourse, and even homosexual behaviour. Divorce, too, is easier to obtain. But society has not by any means lowered all the barriers. As a rule contraceptives and advice about them for the married are not yet supplied free, although the necessary "medical grounds" are becoming thinner; for the unmarried girl they are difficult to obtain but becoming easier; sheaths are freely displayed in chemist's shops and at the barber's, but they are not to be seen in slot machines where they might be obtained in the evenings after these shops have shut.

The argument between those who welcome these changes and those for whom they are the scent of decay in society can be re-phrased. In essence it is between those people who believe in an absolute moral law which should govern all men in all societies and those who say that moral laws arise from the needs of a society at any one time; if the needs change dramatically, as has happened in developed countries in this century, moral attitudes must change too or that society will have shown itself to be incapable of adaptation.

Religious leaders are in a greater difficulty than others who lead and mould opinion. Their law, dependent as it is on the written word, must be immutable. The limits of reinterpretation cannot be very wide. Most churches have, however, managed to adapt themselves in some fashion, if only tacitly, to the menace of exploding populations and the excess of fertility and the only possibly accept-able remedy—birth control. The Roman Catholic church, faced with the prohibition contained in the Pope's encyclical *Humanae Vitae*, remains the exception and is officially and overtly opposed. From the response so far it seems to risk forfeiting the loyalty of the laity and of many priests.

Abortion

Contraception serves the dual purposes of population control and the liberation of the individual from the bonds of excessive fertility. The same can be said of abortion. But abortion necessitates destruc-tion of life and therefore introduces additional and serious social, moral, and religious problems. Virtually all societies have laws on the subject of varying degrees of stringency. At one extreme are the countries whose policy is dominated by the Roman Catholic Church, in most of which abortion is all but totally banned; at the other are Russia, and from time to time other countries, where it is available on medical, eugenic and social grounds so wide as almost to amount to reasons of convenience.

Medicine is intricately involved in the subject because its advances have been partly responsible for the crisis of population expansion that extensive abortion has in some places aimed at overcoming. Other medical advances have so transformed the outlook in a succes-sion of diseases—diabetes, mitral stenosis, hypertension, tuberculosis for example—that patients with them can now have children without serious risk. The medical indications for termination of pregnancy are therefore now predominantly psychiatric. Doctors are citizens and as anxious as anyone else that the laws should be obeyed. Yet it is precisely in psychiatry that definitions of such terms as "danger to health" are most difficult to agree upon. Doctors, too, are often the people to whom the unwillingly pregnant woman first turns; indeed, as often as not, they are the people who first establish the fact that she is pregnant. They see the distress; they may know the effect that an unwanted pregnancy will have on others; they can guess the effect that being unwanted may have on the child as it grows up. Lastly, in the case of a legal abortion—and this is too often slurred over or forgotten—they do the killing, or they carry the responsibility of concurring in it. This is the reverse of their accustomed role.

Undoubtedly a liberalisation of abortion laws does contribute to what Professor Sir Dugald Baird[1] has called the fifth freedom.

[1] Baird, Dugald. (1965), *Brit Med. J.*, **ii,** 1141.

Without doubt, too, abortion, legal and illegal, contributes to population control. Between 1949 and 1959 Japan succeeded in reducing the birth-rate from 34 to 18 per 1,000 by a programme which included abortion, sterilisation, and the encouragement of family planning. About 50% of pregnancies were aborted and the number of legal abortions rose from a quarter of a million in 1949 to over 1,100,000 in 1954. The operation was available on demand and the cost was kept very low (about 6s.).[1] In spite of the popularity of legal operations clandestine operations persisted and it is said that equal numbers of these were done.

In Russia there have been several changes of policy since the revolution.[2] Until 1920 abortion was illegal even on medical grounds. In that year it was made legal on liberal medical and medico-social grounds so long as the operation was performed in hospital. In Moscow by 1926 25,000 legal abortions were done yearly. This figure compares with 65,000 live births in the same year. Mortality from the operation at 0·74 per 1,000 contrasts with a figure of "up to 4%" for illegal abortions. These were reduced to a small fraction according to official figures, which in such matters are, however, never very reliable. In 1936 abortion was prohibited unless continuation of pregnancy constituted a serious threat to life and health. This act was repealed in 1955 because of the alarming rise in the number of illegal operations being done. The repeal was not accompanied by publicity and the main motive does not seem to have been to help population control.

In other countries of Eastern Europe legal abortion has become commonplace: in Hungary more than 150,000 operations a year were done from 1960–63; in Yugoslavia 85,000 a year in 1960–61.

The Scandinavian countries, Sweden, Denmark and Finland, have had the longest experience of the working of liberal laws. "Fifth freedom", eugenics, and health in an extended sense have always been the motive rather than population control. Swedish law allows abortion on the usual medical grounds of danger to physical and mental health. The extensions consist of some rather strictly defined medico-social, humanitarian (pregnancy resulting from rape and coercion or in those below the age of consent, or in the mentally disordered), and eugenic grounds. These acts are administered by medical boards, which shoulder the responsibility for termination. In the early 1950s the therapeutic abortion-rate had risen to about 50 per 1,000 live births, a figure which if transferred to Britain would

[1] Blacker, C. P. (1956). *Eugen. Rev.*, **48**, 30.
[2] Field, M. G. (1956), *New England J. Med.*, **255**, 421.

entail more than 40,000 operations a year. As elsewhere, and to the surprise of many people, a liberal policy has not reduced the number of illegal operations. In Stockholm the percentage of pregnancies legally terminated has varied between 4% and 10% in the period 1947–65. Nevertheless in these years 8% to 11% of pregnancies have ended in criminal abortion.[1] In 1961 Professor Ekblad[2] followed up 255 women five or six years after operation. Generally the patients were very satisfied and there were few serious symptoms afterwards: however, 7% regretted the operation and continued to be disturbed by it. Of these many were childless.

In Britain, attempts to liberalise the abortion laws were made with varying degrees of determination for fifty years before they were successful in 1967. Each new piece of publicity—for instance, the Bourne case in 1937, prison sentences on abortionists, deaths of women after an abortion by unqualified people—strengthened the reformers' purpose. But perhaps the strongest support for their case came from the thalidomide disaster. If the broken-doll appearance of those small children provoked the stricter control of new drugs, it also moved popular opinion in Britain in favour of abortion law reform. The thought that a woman with a probably damaged foetus might be refused a legal abortion, together with, at the election of 1964, the return of a party favourably disposed to reform, gave a new impetus towards clarifying and extending the law.

Even so, the acceptance of the proposed reform by Parliament was more than once in the balance. A strong rearguard action was fought both by those who opposed all abortion—except when the mother's life was at risk—on grounds of conscience and by the conservative members of the medical profession, who refuse to admit that medicine cannot divorce itself today from social issues. Abortion is an unpleasant alternative to contraception for those who do not want to bear a child. Yet as a profession doctors have been singularly reluctant to accept responsibility for giving contraceptive advice.

In the event the Abortion Act, which came into force on 27 April, 1968, allows termination of pregnancy, not only because of feared abnormality of the foetus, but also if its continuance would involve greater risk than termination itself to the life or health of the woman or to her existing children. In deciding the extent of the risk a doctor may take account of her actual or reasonably foreseeable environment. Even before the new law some doctors would openly, and at the cost of the health service, carry out abortions for any of the

[1] Huldt, L. (1968), *Lancet*, **i**, 467.
[2] Ekblad, M. (1961), *Acta Psychiat. Scand.*, supplement 161.

G

reasons now specified. Others would do so less openly and for fees, but with the necessary second opinion in case they were challenged by the police. It remains to be seen whether the effect of the new Act, with its stipulation that abortions must be carried out in health service hospitals or hospitals and nursing homes approved by the Minister of Health, will be to transfer abortions from the second category to the first and, as in Sweden, to leave a great many abortions, still not permitted by the law, to be undertaken illegally and in the back street. There is certainly a possibility that a big rise in demand for abortions could place too great a load on the gynaecologists who are willing to perform the operation. Many are not—and the new Act has a conscience clause to excuse them. Nor do many gynaecologists wish to create the impression that they are too ready to perform the operation lest they find themselves overwhelmed to the detriment of their other more professionally interesting and rewarding work.

These patients at present occupy a bed for from two to five days. A demand for 40,000 operations a year—a likely figure—would need the full time use of 500 hospital beds, without allowing for an unknown number saved by the forestalling of illegal abortions and maternities, that can ill be spared. But technical advance could come to the rescue. In Eastern Europe the aspiration (suction) technique has proved quick, safe and satisfactory in pregnancies of up to twelve weeks.[1] Some British gynaecologists are evaluating this method.

Sterilisation

As it entails no destruction of life and as it is more certain than other methods, sterilisation would seem to be an efficient and acceptable means of contraception. But the situation is far from simple; in some ways it is even more complicated than in other areas where medicine, social policy, religion, and law overlap. For one thing, the public is still very prone to confuse sterilisation with castration and to suppose that, particularly in men, it will damage sexual function. For another, compulsory operations that used to be done in some states of the United States for eugenic reasons, and the Nazi sterilisation law of 1933, have given the operation a bad name. In each case the operation is simple and in theory, if not always in practice, reversible.

No one, apart from Roman Catholics, denies that there are therapeutic indications for sterilisation. These are roughly the same as for abortion, but, as no destruction of a live foetus is involved, many

[1] Dvořák, Z., Trnka, V. and Vašíček, R. (1967), *Lancet*, **ii**, 997.

gynaecologists are more liberal in their interpretation of what constitutes a "threat to health". Naturally there are very few indications for the operation in men, but logically if there are medical indications for a wife to have no more children it would be as satisfactory and simpler to sterilise her husband.

Sterilisation as a measure of contraception, as a more certain, less expensive, and trouble-free form of birth control, is beset with difficulties. There are the usual religious problems and moreover the state of the law is uncertain. The legality of this type of sterilisation has never been properly tested in the courts in Britain. Both Professor Glanville Williams[1] and Mr St John Stevas[2] consider that sterilisation for personal convenience is probably illegal, but since 1966 the Medical Defence Union[3] has been telling doctors that so long as there is full and valid consent the operation is probably legal. The remaining doubt about legality and deep castration fears probably explain why so few operations on men have been done in Britain.

As a means of population control the operation has been used in many countries on both sexes. But if only because it needs doctors to perform it there is doubt about whether it can ever be more than an auxiliary method. In Japan, for example, at a time when over a million abortions were performed in a year, only 38,000 sterilisations took place.[4] In the nine years up to 1957, however, over half a million couples had been protected by sterilisation, by operation on the wife in six out of seven cases. By 1954 in Puerto Rico with its explosive population problem 6% of women in the reproductive ages had been sterilised.[5] India, too, has encouraged sterilisation on a large scale— the figure of 200,000 operations on males has been quoted.[6] In the United States there is evidence[7] that in 1955 1,200,000 people, mainly women, in the reproductive age-group had been sterilised at some time, and further that 45,000 men seek the operation each year.[8] In the face of these substantial figures it is worth remembering that of the organised religions the Roman Catholic, Jewish, Moslem and Buddhist all disapprove of sterilisation.

---

[1] Williams, G. *The Sanctity of Life and the Criminal Law.* (Faber and Faber. London, 1958).
[2] Stevas, N. St J. *Life, Death and the Law.* (Eyre and Spottiswoode. London, 1961).
[3] Addison, P. H. (1966), *Brit. Med. J.* **i,** 1597.
[4] Blacker, C. P. (1956), *Eugen, Rev.,* **48,** 30.
[5] Back, K. W., Hill, R. and Stycos, J. M. (1960). *Law and Contemporary Problems.* **25,** 3. Duke University.
[6] The *Guardian,* 19 July, 1967 said that 2 million operations had been carried out in India in the last two years (90% on men) and that there was a move to make the operation compulsory for those who had had three or more children.
[7] Tietze, C. (1960), *Law and Contemporary Problems.*
[8] Campbell, A. A. (1964), *Amer. J. Obstet. Gynec.,* **89,** 694.

Contraception

Fewer social, religious, and legal complications are associated with contraceptive practices. Indeed in its newest forms, the Pill and the IUCD, contraception is looked on as a saviour of the world in its present and future population crisis.

The drawback of the older methods was that they were so inefficient. Failure-rates per 100 woman-years have been quoted as follows:

Rhythm method   18
Withdrawal   16
Diaphragm (cap) 14·4
Sheath   13·8

Nevertheless, a survey carried out in Britain for the Population Investigation Committee[1] shows that in the 1950s 70% of couples used birth control methods at some time; the figures ranged from 61% in the semi-skilled and unskilled to 80% in the non-manual social classes; of those who were frank about the methods used half preferred the sheath, which had maintained its popularity in spite of the slow growth of methods employed by the female.

The Pill consists of a mixture of sex hormones. One fraction is an oestrogen—the other is a progestogen; the combined effect is to upset the natural negative feedback mechanism between the pituitary and the ovary so that ovulation is inhibited. The essential discovery made by Dr Gregory Pincus and his colleagues in the early 1950s was that recently developed progesterone-like derivatives, which were highly active when given by mouth, could, with oestrogen, be used for this purpose. Clinical use was pioneered by Dr John Rock.

The first of these Pills was marketed in 1955. The convention is to give the Pill once a day for twenty-one days in each month, but this régime is dictated by custom rather than by physiology and the Pill could be taken indefinitely with impunity. It is customary, too, to regard the physiological state as resembling pregnancy but without a foetus in the uterus; a closer parallel would be to temporary castration.

New developments include the giving of the two ingredients in sequence, the possibility of an effective once-a-month pill, and the further possibility of giving a single pill after intercourse to prevent conception.

There are some side-effects, but these are mild and the great

[1] Lafitte, F. *Family Planning and Family Planning Clinics Today*. A survey by the F.P.A. Working Party. Social Study Dept. Birmingham University. (1962).

majority of women experience few of them and can tolerate them easily—nausea, headache, tenderness of the breasts, water-retention, abdominal cramps, depression and loss of libido are some of the commonest—but, to reiterate, they are usually mild. There is no convincing evidence after nine years of any long-term damage to the ovaries, the pituitary, or the liver, nor of any tendency of the Pill to lead to cancer. As for later fertility, of eighty-five women in one survey who had been taking the Pill and then wanted to start a baby, sixty-eight had already conceived within two months of stopping the Pill. Most anxiety has concerned a few women who have suffered from thrombosis and from embolism. These episodes, of course, occasionally happen in women of this age who are not taking the Pill. Much research has gone into this question both in the United States and in Britain and the verdict so far is reassuring. A conference in Chicago and the Food and Drug Administration both exonerated these drugs; one very experienced authority[1] reported not one case in over 5,000 patients. In Britain the Dunlop Committee on the Safety of Drugs[2] found no evidence that the number of women taking the Pill who died in a year from this cause—16—differed significantly from chance expectation—13. In any case the risk of thrombosis from taking the Pill is less than the risk in pregnancy.[3] Nevertheless one out of every 2,000 women on the Pill suffers from thrombo-embolic disease each year. As a contraceptive measure the Pill is highly successful. The failure (pregnancy) rate per 100 woman years ranges from about 0·3 to 3·0 in various reported studies, the majority being below 1·0.

It is in very wide use. Estimates of about a million women taking it in Britain and 5 million in the United States in 1965 are probably not very wide of the mark. Elsewhere it is being increasingly widely used by both educated and unsophisticated people. It was perhaps being taken in 1966 by 7 million women throughout the world.[4] Dr Pincus prescribed it successfully for women in Puerto Rico, and, to quote another champion, "the introduction of oral contraceptives has been highly successful in many parts of Africa. The Pill is aesthetically acceptable . . ."[5] But many people think that it is unsuitable for wide use in regions of the world where supervision is precarious, communications and access to supplies difficult and where there may

[1] Tyler, E. T. (1964). *Brit. Med. J.*, **ii**, 843.
[2] Cahal, D. A. (1965), *Lancet*, **ii**, 1013.
[3] According to the Minister of Health's statement of 4 April, 1967 further research has shown a slightly increased risk of thrombo-embolic disorder but the risk is small and less than that which arises from ordinary pregnancy.
[4] *Medical News.* 1 November, 1966.
[5] Purcell, F. M. (1965), *Brit. Med. J.* **ii**, 1242.

be a language barrier and illiteracy to hinder adequate instruction. The liability of the Pill to produce side-effects, though counter-balanced in some people by a sense of increased well-being and the relief of premenstrual tension, would be all too likely to lead the ill-educated and unsupervised to abandon it readily. For these reasons family planners in India have rejected it so far for widespread use in their programmes.[1]

The intra-uterine contraceptive device has a long history, but there has been an intense revival of interest in it since 1959. It is the successor to the devices used by Gräfenberg over a period of many years between the wars. He employed silkworm gut, or gut strength-ened with silver wire and finally a ring of silver wire. Although he used it successfully others had less happy experiences and it fell into disrepute, particularly in the United States. In some hands the side-effects were serious—cases of perforation and sepsis occurred—and it was spontaneously expelled in 3–4% of people. Nor was it much more successful than simpler and safer methods of contracep-tion. In some reports pregnancy-rates of up to 10 per 100 woman-years were found. Nevertheless it continued to be used, though not widely, and a few gynaecologists had much more encouraging results. Interest revived in the technique with reports from Japan where Dr Ishihama[2] had used the method on 18,000 women, and from Israel where it had been used by Dr Oppenheimer with very satisfactory results on 329 women.[3]

Since then new materials, new techniques of introduction, and a worldwide wealth of experience have generated a new enthusiasm. Three types are in common use, the Lippes loop, the Birnberg bow, and the Margulies spiral. They are all made of polyethylene "wire" (a product of this plastics age) impregnated with radio-opaque material so that their position can, if necessary, be checked by X-rays. They are introduced into the uterus in linear form through a hollow tube with a plunger. Once in the uterus and extruded from the introducer they take up their characteristic shape. No anaesthetic is required.

It is necessary to ensure that the uterus is not abnormal and in particular that the woman is not pregnant. Introduction, for this reason, is best done immediately a period has ended or two months after a confinement. So far as is known there is no reason why the device should not stay in place for an indefinite period but, till more

[1] Austin, G. S. *The Times*, 14 August, 1965.
[2] Ishihama, A. (1959). *Yokohama Med. J.*, **10**, 89.
[3] Oppenheimer, W. (1959), *Amer. J. Obst. and Gynec.*, **78**, 446.

is known, many doctors prefer to remove it for a month every year or two.

The side-effects are few—slight abdominal cramps and one or two heavy periods may be experienced by 10% of women; sepsis is very rare and there is no evidence whatever that the device can cause cancer. Its chief drawbacks are that it can be difficult to insert in women who have not had a baby, and in them side-effects are likely to be more frequent; that the loop or bow or spiral may be extruded in 4 or 5% though reinsertion is often successful; and that up to 4% of women may remove the device themselves because of discomfort. In those who have been successfully fitted pregnancy rates are low—in the region of 3–4 per 100 woman-years.

There are already enthusiastic reports covering many thousands of cases,[1] and the impression gained is that in skilled hands the device is safe, popular and reliable, with few complications and few failures.

There are of course many variables: the skill and experience of the gynaecologist; the intelligence of the population at risk; the efficacy of the device itself. One report,[2] for example, recounted the experiences of 2,906 insertions in which one of the bows used had a failure (pregnancy) rate of 12·4 per 100 woman-years. This author has abandoned insertions in those who have had no children because of the high risk of spontaneous expulsion and the frequency of side-effects. It is probably too early yet to be sure that it is going to be wholly satisfactory, particularly as there is no firm knowledge of how it works. The IUCD's special virtues are its cheapness—a fraction of a penny—and its once-for-all character. The woman who has been successfully fitted only needs to do anything positive if she wants to have a baby. The Indian authorities' initial enthusiasm has, however, been tempered by a disappointing response from Indian women to the campaign to fit as many women as possible with the device.

A rough balance sheet has been struck in Table 4 on the next page. One inference to be drawn from this table is that a couple might be wise to use the Pill until after their first child has been born and then the IUCD. When they are sure that they want no more children the husband might be sterilised. It is high time that the law on contraceptive sterilisation was clarified.

An ironic postscript to this discussion of population problems and their possible solutions ought perhaps to be recorded. Such are the vagaries of human fertility that one and the same branch of

---

[1] Tietze, C. and Lewit, S. *Proceedings of the Population Council Conference on Intra-uterine Contraceptive Devices.* Excerpta Medica Foundation. (New York, 1964).
[2] Hall, R. E. (1966), *Amer. J. Obst. and Gynec.,* **94,** 1.

TABLE 4

Three large-scale methods of contraception compared.

	Pill	IUCD	Sterilisation of males
Length of experience in use	since early 1950s	since 1959	centuries
Reliability	99%	95%	100%
Number of people unsuitable	Few	Many	None
Side-effects	Fairly common	Less common	None
Further attendance	Frequent	Infrequent	Unnecessary
Expenditure of skilled time	Much	Little	Little
Cost	High	Low	Low
Language barrier a problem	Yes	Little	Little
Reversible	100%	100%	40%
Difficulties about acceptability	None	Little	Much more

the medical profession—sometimes perhaps the same person—is involved in artificial insemination and the other means of helping the infertile, in efforts to combat perinatal mortality, in sterilisation of women, in prescribing pills and fitting devices for contraception, and in therapeutic abortion.

These are fields too in which medical education has been slow to catch up with human needs. In some of them public opinion is pressing action on a reluctant profession.

Population Quality

Faced with the need to control and limit the absolute number of their populations, faced with the prospect of starvation, the under-developed countries have not, or at least not yet, concerned themselves with population quality. But in the West there has been fear that the combined effect of medicine's success in keeping people alive and the use of contraception is dysgenic. The more intelligent section of the population, it is argued, limit their families; the unskilled, the unintelligent, and the unfit do not, or do so less efficiently. Yet they no longer experience a high death rate to do it for them.

The argument, transferred to the world scale, is similar to that used by nationalists and racialists for encouraging more births in their own countries.

To some this crude eugenic argument seems axiomatic. But its simplicity is deceptive. What is the evidence? Whereas the problems of population size can be analysed on a firm foundation of facts and figures, in the question of quality there is a morass of ignorance, speculation, assertion and imprecision, made worse, moreover, by the ideological mists of the nature *vs* nurture controversy.

Is the national intelligence falling? That in this difficult field things are not always what they seem to be is well illustrated by alarm over the trend of the national intelligence. At the time of the investigations of Britain's Royal Commission on Population in 1944–48 it was firmly established that there was a negative correlation between intelligence and size of family. This was, in Britain, of the order of 0·2–0·25. Many eminent authorities in this subject also agreed that there was evidence of a fall of about two I.Q. points between one generation and the next. As Sir Cyril Burt[1] pointed out this would mean that the numbers of children of scholarship ability would be halved in fifty years and the number of the feeble-minded almost doubled.

This evidence and the weight of authority seemed very convincing, but one of these authorities, Professor Sir Godfrey Thomson,[2] who had said in his Galton Lecture, "In short, the educational system of the country acts as a sieve to sift out the more intelligent and destroy their posterity", produced in 1948 some new and weighty evidence to confound his earlier views. A group intelligence test was given in 1947 to virtually all eleven year-olds in Scotland similar to one that had been given to children in the same age-group in 1932. The results amply confirmed the expectation of a negative correlation between total score and family size in 1947 as in 1932. But between these years the mean score, far from falling, had risen 1·3 I.Q. points for boys and 3·2 points for girls.[3]

Most authorities attributed this surprising result to test sophistication, to improved nutrition, or to better teaching, in accordance with their personal choice. Since then, however, little has been heard from the pessimists. One reason may be that it is probable that since the war differential fertility is much less apparent. It may perhaps even be in the process of becoming reversed. Nevertheless the question is not yet disposed of.

Eugenics, Positive and Negative

The classic Galtonian remedy for diseases and defects known to be hereditary is popularly supposed to be "to check the birth rate of the

[1] Burt, Sir C. *Intelligence and Fertility.* Occasional Papers on Eugenics. (Eugenics Society and Hamish Hamilton Medical Books. London, 1946).
[2] Thomson, Sir G. *The Trend of National Intelligence.* Occasional Papers on Eugenics. (1946).
[3] *The Trend of Scottish Intelligence.* (London, 1949).

unfit, instead of allowing them to come into being . . ." It is seldom recalled that Galton laid equal, sometimes more, stress on positive eugenics—"the improvement of the race by furthering the productivity [sic] of the fit by early marriages and healthful rearing of their children."[1]

It cannot be said that we have got very far yet with positive eugenic policies, if only because so many of the "desirable qualities" are a matter of personal opinion and because the genetic component in them is so questionable. At least social policies tend towards enabling gifted children, like others, to develop their full potential. It is far easier, too, for the intelligent to marry before they have finished training, to marry early, and thus to have larger families.

Negative eugenics, on the other hand, has run into difficulties. The "unfit"—those with genetic handicaps—have been more clearly distinguished from the merely unfortunate; modes of inheritance have been more accurately defined; and the fact has been recognised that non-specific dullness and subnormality, as opposed to most of the named varieties, derive genetically from numerous genes, each of which has only a small effect. To sterilise the subnormal can make some eugenic sense, but as these genes and many recessive genes are so widely distributed in the population it is difficult to agree with one authority who says: "the eugenic prevention of mental deficiency undoubtedly remains the chief hope for the future, and in no other way can we expect any large-scale effect."[2] The sterilisation of the subnormal can make more social sense if, as is so often the case, they are incapable of bringing up children properly.

It has been calculated by Professor Penrose[3] that if two normal people have already produced a feeble-minded child the chance that the next child will be similar is 8 in 100; but if both parents are dull themselves the chance of the next child being feeble-minded is almost 1 in 2. Sterilisation, if the genes concerned are multiple or recessive, will be eugenic in the immediate sense, but to expect any substantial degree of racial improvement by such means is mistaken. Professor Fisher, for example, estimated many years ago[4] that only 11% of the feeble-minded came from feeble-minded parents.

The whole theory of negative eugenics has been questioned by some geneticists. Their view is that we do not understand at all completely how natural selection operates in the human race. Apparently "bad" genes, like those responsible for some varieties of

[1] Blacker, C. P. *Eugenics: Galton and After*. (Duckworth. London, 1952).
[2] Mayer-Gross, W., Slater, E. and Roth, M. *Clinical Psychiatry*. (Cassell. London, 1954).
[3] Penrose, L. S. (1939), *Eugen. Rev.*, **31**, 35.
[4] Fisher, R. A. (1927), *J. Heredity*, **18**, 529.

mental defect, may take part in a genetic equilibrium, their disadvantages being balanced by some other compensating advantage such as increased fertility. The most obvious example of compensation is the sickle-cell trait. This gene confers on its possessor an abnormal haemoglobin. If he is homozygous for this trait (that is, has inherited it from both parents) he is likely to die of sickle-cell anaemia in childhood; if he is heterozygous (inherited from one parent only) some of his haemoglobin will be abnormal and he is likely to experience only some mild symptoms from time to time.

Following hints and speculations in earlier work Dr Allison established[1] in 1954 that these heterozygotes were more resistant to subtertian malaria than other people who had only normal haemoglobin A. There had to be some such advantage possessed by these heterozygotes to explain how the gene had maintained itself at such a high frequency in certain populations in spite of its rapid elimination through death from sickle-cell anaemia. In parts of Africa 20%, and in parts of Greece 17%, of the population possessed this sickling trait.

There are other examples of apparently bad genes being not wholly bad, but this is the most conspicuous case so far identified. A corollary of this view is that these genes help to maintain the diversity of the whole pool of human genetic material available for recombination in successive generations. They help populations to avoid the dangers of in-breeding, uniformity of hereditary material and lack of variance. Sir Ronald Fisher[2] called this variance the "energy" of the species, and Professor Penrose, who clearly approves of this view, has said: "Given sufficient energy, the human race should be able, even without the aid of eugenics, to adapt itself biologically to civilised life without risking extinction."[3]

If one accepts these propositions that not all apparently bad genes are wholly bad, and that differential fertility may mask a state of equilibrium, there is still room for some apprehension about the effects of medicine on population quality. By our efforts the genetic equilibrium is altered. There must be a genetic component even in infectious disease, an inherited variation in susceptibility to infection. The successful chemotherapy of tuberculosis, for example, preserves the more susceptible and their genes, so that in time they must become more frequent in the population. Perhaps this case of preservation does not have so harmful an effect as it would in other

[1] Allison, A. C. (1954), *Brit. Med. J.* **i,** 290.
[2] Fisher, R. A. *The Genetical Theory of Natural Selection.* (Clarendon Press. Oxford, 1930).
[3] Penrose, L. S. *The Biology of Mental Defect.* (Sidgwick and Jackson. London, 1949).

infections. Any increase in susceptibility to tuberculous infection may well be balanced by other consequences of medical advance: the more susceptible, for example, are less likely nowadays to come in contact with a dose of organisms sufficient to infect them; if they do the illness can be identified early and treated effectively.

With illness in which the genetic component is more obvious, the potentially harmful effects of therapy on the genetic constitution of the population is clear even if the effect on the individual is beneficial or life-saving. The infant with congenital hypertrophic pyloric stenosis who is saved by surgical operation, the phenylketonuric who is saved from an institutional life by early diagnosis and a phenylalanine-free diet, the young diabetic who survives many years with treatment, can all later have children. In time these and other diseases like them must increase in frequency. So will the need for treating them. Of this ill-effect Professor Darlington[1] has said: "all medically and surgically curable genetic defects, we can predict, will therefore increase in populations enjoying the full advantages of medical and surgical treatment. Unless, that is, the community, or the medical profession, or the individuals concerned, aware of what is happening, that is of the genetic principles concerned, take steps to avoid the disastrous consequences of their own achievements."

Remedies

On the assumption that there are grounds for anxiety, that medical science is preserving too many of the unfit, what should be done about it? Can we rely on the voluntary birth control of the unfit to redress the balance? As eugenic measures birth control methods are so far making slow headway. Some countries have eugenic laws, compulsory or more often permissive. But the whole trend of the times is away from compulsion; opinion is strongly influenced by the liberal view that there have to be very strong grounds indeed for removing a person's right to have children. Much more reliance is being placed on voluntary sterilisation, but there are two difficulties. How valid is the consent from a subnormal person? How valid, too, is consent obtained under the duress implicit in such a situation as: "if you have the operation you may go home or have spells of leave from hospital; or be released from prison sooner." Today sterilisation is seldom done for eugenic reasons. More often the reasons are economic or social.

[1] Darlington, C. D. *Genetics and Man*. (George Allen and Unwin. London, 1964).

One recent technical advance, if it develops in the next few years, might make eugenic abortion more acceptable. It is now possible to culture cells obtained from human amniotic fluid.[1] These cells are derived from the foetal skin and kidney and they can be subjected to chromosome analysis.[2] Thus, not only can the sex of the foetus be established but chromosomal abnormalities can also be detected—mongolism is the obvious example. The twentieth week is at present unfortunately the earliest time that this investigation can be done. If such a foetus could be identified earlier, a eugenic therapeutic abortion, performed on the basis of this kind of evidence, would be acceptable to public opinion.

As a eugenic measure contraception is largely free of so many of the objections attaching to sterilisation and abortion. No doubt as it becomes more certain, as is already happening, it will be more exclusively employed. The slow spread of genetic counselling clinics is encouraging. From these, people who have specific problems can get accurate advice. Should a woman have children if the husband's uncle has Huntington's chorea? If a couple's first child is severely subnormal, what are the chances that further children will be affected? A diabetic girl wants to marry a man whose mother also has the disease—should she have children? Can heterozygotes for various recessive genes be identified? These are the kind of questions. The answers may be unhappy, and they are often irritatingly statistical, but they can be the basis for rational decisions. Coupled with contraception this sort of advice could succeed in removing most of the objectionable prickles from negative eugenics.

Biological Discovery

On the other tack positive eugenists, if they have learned lessons from the storms that negative eugenists have run into, will have to keep a sharp look-out. Biological science has advanced so fast and so far that experiments in human breeding could be made of such a far-reaching nature that the ensuing social, legal, ethical and religious consequences would make the rumpus about artificial insemination from a donor seem like a storm in a teacup. Sperms can be preserved for years and remain active; fertilised ova can be implanted in a different individual animal and grow; before long it may be possible to grow human reproductive cells in tissue culture and to alter genetic material deliberately to breed special characteris-

[1] Fuchs, F. and Riis, P. (1956). *Nature*, **177**, 330.
[2] Steel, M. W. and Breg, W. R. (1966), *Lancet*, **i**, 383.

tics. True "test-tube babies" are still beyond the horizon and human life synthesised from simple materials even farther away. Within the next few years, however, society and medicine will probably have to reckon with the possibility of a child being born to a woman that originated in an egg from another woman and a sperm from a man perhaps long dead.

At the cellular and molecular level biological discoveries in exciting and feverish succession have so far had remarkably little practical effect on medicine. This is not to decry them. There must always be a gap between the discoveries of pure science and their application to human use for good or ill. In atomic physics it took thirty years or so for fundamental discoveries about the atom to flower not only in atom-bombs but also in nuclear power stations, radio-isotopes and vast machines for the treatment of cancer. In cellular and micro and molecular biology we are in that gap now. It was only in 1944 that it was proved that[1] bacterial transformation depended on the transfer of deoxyribonucleic acid (DNA) from one strain to another, and that this material embodied the genetic information in each cell; and only in 1953 was the Watson-Crick model of the structure of DNA, which illustrated how self-replication might occur, proposed. Already our fundamental concepts have been transformed: a gene is the capacity to make an enzyme; a virus is a particle of infectious heredity; the distinction between living and non-living matter has evaporated; the specificity of a gene lies in the arrangement rather than in the composition of its constituents—to mention just a few. But the breakthroughs are in the future—the control of virus infection, a cure for cancer, a solution to the problems of immunity—and when they come they are all likely to emerge from this branch of science. The dangers are there too: first, the possibility raised by Sir Macfarlane Burnet[2] of the escape from a laboratory of an exceptionally virulent virus to which no one has any immunity, or of the unlimited spread of a cancer-producing virus, with alarming applications to bacteriological warfare; secondly, and even more menacing, the creation of artificial life from simple materials—at the moment a figment of science fiction.

Meanwhile the practical value of all this research has been limited. Clinical observation has so far been of more use than experimental work in the field of chemotherapy and the resistance of bacteria to antibiotics. But pure research and technical advances at the cellular level have established, it seems surprisingly late in the day, that

Avery, O. T., McLeod, C. M. and McCarty, M. (1944), *J. Experimental Med.*, **79,** 137.
[2] Burnet, F. M. (1966), *Lancet*, **i,** 37.

human cells contain twenty-three pairs of chromosomes. Now that they can be seen under the microscope and individually identified and numbered, a succession of rare anomalies of chromosome number, size and shape has been linked to clinical syndromes— mongolism, various peculiarities of the sex chromosomes and several others. This elegant work chiefly concerns some rather rare causes of mental subnormality. It has elucidated the cause of some very rare types of intersex. Perhaps it will soon illuminate some causes of criminality. It is disappointing but not surprising that it has failed to shed any light at all on the causes of homosexuality.

Biological discoveries may have opened up new horizons in genetics and shown how, in the future, the quality of human populations can be controlled. Perhaps the newest branch of biological science— gerontology—will in the near future prove as fruitful in discovering how the process of ageing can be delayed. It is time to turn from the question of quality and the problem of numbers to consider the advanced countries and their ageing populations.

CHAPTER SIX

Population Problems II: Ageing Populations

Much has been said in earlier chapters about the causes of the fall in mortality in advanced countries. One cannot do better than to quote Professor McKeown[1] again in order to hammer home the point: ". . . in order of relative importance the main influences responsible for the decline in mortality . . . have been: a rising standard of living; the control of the physical environment; and specific preventive and curative therapy."

In our century, especially in the last forty years, personal health services and specific therapy have played a more and more important part. The results have been that mortality has fallen, particularly among the young—see Chart I (p. 45); that more people survive into old age; and that in old age thanks to a hundred and one medical measures—and social measures too—chronic diseases, deformities, disabilities and handicaps abound.

Tables 3 and 2 have shown how diabetics and the tuberculous now survive into old age. People suffering from a host of other medical conditions survive too. Hence the specialty of geriatrics; hence the new science of gerontology; hence psycho-geriatrics; and hence, too, a preoccupation with the quality of a life prolonged excessively, and renewed interest in euthanasia.

The Fall in Mortality of the Young

In Britain today 70% of deaths occur at the age of sixty-five or more. This is twice the corresponding figure forty years ago. People now die predominantly in old age.

Chart III and Table 5 (p.114) show some of the changes that have occurred in the age distribution and the mortality of the population of England and Wales in this century. Percentages and rates have been used to clarify the trends because the total population has increased by one-third in this time.

[1] McKeown, T. *Medicine in Modern Society.*

Less than half of the population is now under thirty-five; in 1921 the figure was three-fifths. In the same period the proportion of the population which is sixty-five years old or more has doubled. The numbers of the extremely old—those who are eighty-five or more— have multiplied four and a half times. It has been forecast[1] that in the next fifteen years the number of people who are over sixty-five will increase by another 27%.

Age–distribution of the population in different years   Chart III

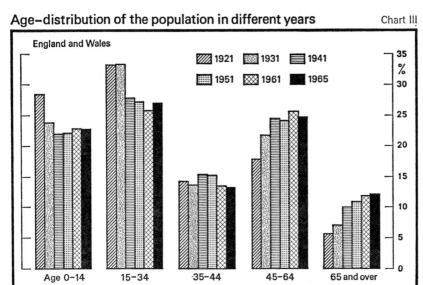

Source: Registrar General's Statistical Reviews. Part 1. Tables, medical. Table 1

In spite of an increase of one-fifth in the population between 1921 and 1961 the number of deaths in each age-group decreased until the age of fifty-five. Before the age of thirty-five only about one-fifth as many died. If death rates are calculated on the basis of the number of people in each age group living (Table 5) the figures are equally impressive.

Death rates have fallen steeply in childhood and early adult life. In planning a family parents of today no longer have to expect that one or more of their children will not survive into adult life. In each year between the ages of five and nine, for example, only four children in every 10,000 will die. Knowledge of this sort must be an important element in our confidence that we can control our environment. This fall in mortality is mainly a consequence of the control of infectious disease. In the age groups 0–44 deaths from these diseases fell from

[1] *The Population of Britain*. Central Office of Information. R5616. (London, 1964).

H

TABLE 5

Death rates per 1000 living in age-groups.
England and Wales.

Year	Infant Mortality*	1—	5—	10—	15—	20—	25—	35—	45—	55—	65—	75—	85—
1901–05	138		3·74	2·19	3·11	4·00	5·44	8·86	14·9	28·7	59·4	127·3	258·6
1911–15	110		3·39	2·08	2·88	3·58	4·57	7·28	13·1	26·2	57·3	126·2	257·9
1921–25	76		2·48	1·71	2·61	3·30	3·79	5·71	10·1	21·6	51·1	121·8	251·4
1931–35	62	6·56	2·18	1·41	2·33	2·96	3·20	4·82	9·44	20·1	49·0	119·3	255·7
1941–45	50	3·50	1·50	1·08	1·96	3·06	3·04	3·95	8·00	18·1	43·0	104·5	213·0
1950	30	1·35	0·64	0·48	0·90	1·24	1·57	2·62	6·72	17·0	42·7	106·9	227·6
1955	25	1·00	0·43	0·38	0·64	0·86	1·10	2·23	6·14	16·1	41·4	105·1	233·5
1960	22	0·87	0·44	0·32	0·64	0·81	0·93	2·07	5·73	15·6	38·8	97·0	217·3
1965	19	0·82	0·40	0·36	0·70	0·75	0·88	2·14	5·83	15·6	38·3	92·5	209·9

Source: Registrar General's Statistical Review for 1965.
Part I. Table 4

*per 1,000
live births

40,000 in 1930 to 866 in 1965. But to apportion the credit is even more difficult than it was for the similar changes in the nineteenth century, if only because there are more candidates to share it.

To record these impressive figures of changing mortality is not to imply that infectious diseases have ceased to be important. They are, after all, in the form of upper respiratory infection still the commonest reason for people to consult a doctor. Problems of altered virulence and of drug resistance still need watching and cross infection and the hospital staphylococcus still kill people. Alarm has been expressed,[1] too, about the drastic reduction in the number of beds available in Britain for cases of infectious disease and the shortage of trained nurses and doctors to staff them.

One consequence of the decline in mortality has been that doctors and research workers have been left freer to tackle the other causes of death and disease in childhood and early adult life. The congenital malformations have in some cases been shown to have environmental causes (maternal rubella, thalidomide, folic acid deficiency and some cases of maternal diabetes); studies have been made of the causes of prematurity and units for the special care of premature babies are common. A great deal of research has gone into the prevention and treatment of haemolytic disease of the newborn, which is caused by an incompatibility between the rhesus blood factors of the parents. Many centres are now equipped to give affected newborn infants exchange transfusions, and a few for injecting blood into the peritoneal cavity of a still unborn infant who is likely to be severely affected.[2][3][4]—a remarkable technical feat. Exchange transfusion, while the baby is still within the uterus, has even been performed.[5][6]

Indeed, intense study of the foetus before and just after birth, its genetics, biochemistry and physiology, its interaction with the pre-natal environment and the cold world afterwards, and its diseases, is a new field for medicine. It will need a new name—embryonics perhaps.

For children between the ages of one and fourteen accident is now the commonest cause of death. Many of these accidents happen in the home from burns and scalds and from swallowing tablets that have been left about within reach. Although these deaths are readily

[1] Ramsey, A. M., Emond, R. T. D. and Alston, J. M. (1964), *Brit. Med. J.*, **ii**, 1004.
[2] Liley, A. W. (1963), *Brit. Med. J.*, **ii**, 1107.
[3] Holman, C. A. and Karnicki, J. (1964), *Brit. Med. J.*, **ii**, 594.
[4] Holman, C. A. and Karnicki, J. (1966). *Proc. Roy. Soc. Med.*, **59**, 81.
[5] Freda, V. J. and Adamsons, K. (1964), *Amer. J. Obst. and Gynec.*, **89**, 817.
[6] It now seems possible to prevent Rh disease from occurring at all by giving the mother a dose of anti-D gammaglobulin within 48 hours of the birth of a child that might otherwise make her produce Rh antibodies. (Clarke, C. A. 1967, *Brit. Med. J.* **i, iv**, 7.).

preventable many years of persuasion were needed before legislation was enacted to prohibit the sale of inflammable night clothing for children or of gas and electric fires with inadequate guards.

Accidents are the commonest cause of death, too, in the age-group 15–44 and, in theory at any rate, they are preventable. To prevent all risk is obviously impossible. It would impose a ban on swimming, climbing, factory work and, of course, travelling on the roads. Even so, some improvement should be possible; in the age group 15–24 in 1965, for example, more than 40% of the male deaths were caused by motor vehicle traffic accidents.

In middle life cancer, degenerative diseases of the heart and blood vessels and chronic bronchitis declare themselves as successors to tuberculosis as captains of the men of death, a situation that they occupy even more defiantly in old age. These are major unsolved problems in medicine and they pre-empt research and doctors' time to an ever-increasing extent.

One further result of the fading away of infectious disease has been to throw into relief mental illness and subnormality as massive causes of disablement. In the redistribution of interest, time and money that has taken place psychiatry has gained a great deal.

An Ageing Population

A second consequence—and one of vast social significance—is inescapable. Most of those who would have died each year, had the toll of infectious disease continued, live on into middle age, and presumably will survive into old age. What is sometimes forgotten is that the steepest fall in mortality from infectious disease occurred barely twenty years ago. Those who benefited most were below thirty-five years of age. They are still middle-aged or less and the full impact on the numbers of elderly in the population has yet to be felt. In 1961 there were 5·5 million people aged sixty-five or more in England and Wales. It has been estimated that by 1979 there may well be over 7 million. But there could be a pause soon after as those born in the lean years 1925–40 begin to enter the ranks of the elderly.

This trend is not, of course, confined to Great Britain. It is apparent in most of the other countries of Western Europe and in North America. There are 18 million people aged sixty-five or more today, for example, in the United States. It is expected that, by 1975, there will be 20.7 million old people in America out of a total of 221 million—nearly one in ten. Elsewhere, as infectious disease is brought under control, the population must become older unless war, famine or new plagues intervene. One reason for this trend to cause alarm in Britain is that an ageing population, coupled with an increase in the school-leaving age and an extension of tertiary education, has diminished the ratio of the working to the dependent population. Because of the low birth-rate in the years 1925–40, whose cohorts have long since entered the working population, the ratio has become lower still.

Geriatric Medicine

Ageing populations, so characteristic of our time, have brought difficulties to medicine, too, for the elderly, man for man—or more probably woman for woman—are estimated to make three times as great a demand on doctors' time as the working population. Medicine has replied with the creation of a special branch—geriatrics—to study and treat illness in this age group. The name was coined by Ignatz Nascher in the United States in 1909,[1] but interest in the subject did not become at all widespread until just before the 1939–45 war. Since then the specialty has flourished and the number of geriatric physicians has multiplied, although they have not quite established parity of esteem with many of medicine's other specialists. It is as though the aura of the workhouse still envelops them just as memories of the tuberculosis officer and the asylum doctor still cling to the chest physician and the psychiatrist.

Geriatrics did, in fact, begin in the Poor Law infirmaries, which housed the elderly chronic sick; they were regarded as incurable and clinically uninteresting, and were refused admission by general hospitals, including the teaching hospitals, so that no medical students ever saw them. Nor, as a rule, do they today—so slow is the pace of change in Britain's medical schools.

Geriatric medicine has had difficulty in defining its boundaries. For statistical and administrative purposes it would be useful to have the subject linked to an age-group of the population. But here confusion has crept in. Many of the numerous surveys that have been made of the relevant population, such as that by the Nuffield Foundation,[2] [3] concern themselves with men who are sixty-five and over and women who are sixty and more, because these are the ages covered by the Pensions Acts. This definition of old age was also

[1] Nascher, I. (1909), *New York Med. J.*, 21 August.
[2] Rowntree, B. S. *Old People.* Nuffield Foundation. (Geoffrey Cumberlege—Oxford University Press. London, 1947).
[3] Sheldon, J. H. *The Social Medicine of Old Age.* Nuffield Foundation. (Geoffrey Cumberlege—Oxford University Press. London, 1948).

taken in the Phillips report[1] on the financial problems of the provision for old age. Others, however, including the Registrar General
and the Ministry of Health, prefer to regard old age as starting at
sixty-five in both sexes, and this is the group to which most unofficial
publications apply nowadays.

The fact is that medicine and geriatrics need an operative rather
than a statistical definition. Many old people do not suffer from
diseases or disabilities at all; others develop diseases, acute or chronic,
which respond as well to ordinary treatment as in anyone else. In
them, as in younger people, the disease—pneumonia, an exacerba-
tion of chronic bronchitis, a broken leg, or an attack of mental
depression—is an episode. When it is over they return home and
carry on as before. But many present far more complex problems.

Old people may have multiple diseases and disabilities—chronic
bronchitis, a failing heart, arthritis, paralyses, corns and painful
deformed toes, partial blindness and deafness—which restrict their
independence and may confine them to a chair or even to bed for
long periods. A random sample[2] of 200 people of sixty-five and over
in Edinburgh in 1962–63 showed that the men had an average of
3·26 and the women 3·42 physical disabilities. In each case fewer
than half these handicaps were known to their family doctors. Only
22% had no disability or only a slight one. In the United States the
National Health Survey estimated that in 1957–58 only one-quarter
of the men and one-fifth of the women aged sixty-five or more were
free of chronic ailments; almost one-third had three or more.[3] On the
basis of a sample of more than 4,000 elderly people throughout
Britain, Professor Townsend and Mrs Wedderburn[4] have calculated
that 750,000 of the elderly living at home are either permanently in
bed (122,000) or confined to the building where they live.

Old people may also suffer from a degree of mental enfeeblement
or, more seriously, a psychosis either of organic origin—a senile or
arteriosclerotic dementia—or non-organic, of which a severe depression is far the commonest. Many surveys both in Britain and in other
countries have shown that there is much serious mental disorder in
old age that remains untreated. An investigation in Newcastle upon

[1] *Report of the Committee on the Economic and Financial Problems of the Provision for Old Age.*
(H.M.S.O. London, 1954).
[2] Williamson, J., Stokoe, I. H., Gray, S., Fisher, M., Smith, A., McGhee, A. and
Stephenson, E. (1964), *Lancet*, **i**, 1117.
[3] U.S. National Health Survey. *Limitation of Activity and Mobility due to Chronic Conditions.* United States, July, 1957–June, 1958. U.S. Public Health Services Publication
584–B11. (July, 1959). Quoted in *Contemporary Economic Problems and Issues* by Hailstones,
T. J., Martin, B. L. and Wing, G. (South-Western Publishing Co. Cincinnati, Ohio, 1966).
[4] Townsend, P. and Wedderburn, D. *The Aged in the Welfare State.* Occasional Papers
on Social Administration. No.14. (G. Bell. London, 1965).

Tyne into the prevalence of these illnesses[1] found that 10% of those living at home showed mild or severe organic syndromes and a further 30% were found to be suffering from other psychiatric disorders, mainly neuroses. The Edinburgh survey, too, disclosed a reservoir of dementia and other psychiatric illness, most of which was unknown to the family doctors.

There may also be a need among old people for social help, for money, a better diet, more suitable housing, or one or more of a score of social services—chiropody, home nursing, a club to go to, a regular hot meal, laundry service, a home help, regular visiting and occupation. Only about one in eight of these elderly people living at home makes use of any of the local welfare services. Certainly many more need help but are unaware of what aid is available or lack the initiative to seek it.

Many old people come into two or more of these categories, and it is the complexity of the problems that old people so often present that gives geriatrics its *raison d'être*. From the medico-social point of view there is no valid reason why the specialty should be tied to a particular age. Indeed a widow of fifty-nine who lives alone in a top-floor flat and who then suffers a stroke from which she recovers incompletely will become essentially a geriatric problem. But with advancing years, and especially beyond seventy, multiple disabilities are commoner, psychiatric complications creep in, spouses die and more help is needed.

The recurring lessons of all surveys of the state of the elderly are that there is a great deal more physical and psychiatric disability in this age-group of the population than has hitherto been suspected; that by the time they reach hospital the diseases are far advanced and the disabilities long-established; and that there is need for much more social help, which in fact is not given because it is not asked for.

Perhaps the fear of the workhouse and its infirmary and of being "put away" lingers on; ignorance, inertia and ingrained habit certainly play a part. It seems likely that in the case of the old, as for decades with the mentally subnormal and more recently with the incompletely recovered psychotic, the community's health and welfare services (including the general practitioner) will have to pursue illness into people's homes if the burden of ill-health that sits on the elderly is to be discovered and an attempt made to lift it. This will add handsomely to the cost of health services.

Once elderly patients reach him the geriatric physician can often do a great deal. He can diagnose illnesses and treat them; alleviate

[1] Kay, D. W. K., Beamish, P. and Roth M. (1964). *Brit. J. Psychiat*, **110**, 146.

disabilities, arrange for the provision of hearing aids, spectacles and walking aids for those who need them; he can assess the psychiatric needs of the patient, if necessary with the help of a psychiatrist, and arrange for treatment; lastly, with the help of social workers, he can assess the social needs of the patient when she returns home and organise all the forms of help necessary, or if the patient is unfit to go home, determine to what kind of accommodation she ought to be admitted—long-term annexe, day hospital, welfare home, sheltered housing and so forth. The proportion of the elderly over 65 who are in hospitals and homes is at present surprisingly low. According to Professor Townsend's survey[1]—and others agree—only 4·5% (280,000) were in institutions of any kind—of whom 38% were in residential homes, 21% in psychiatric beds, and 41% in other hospitals and nursing homes. The remainder—19 out of 20 old people—were living independent lives. In spite of this, the provision of beds for the elderly who need to be in hospitals and of places in homes is already inadequate. Clearly, with the increase in numbers, unless priority is given to it, the provision will be more inadequate still.

The Townsend survey did not find that, as has often been alleged, people nowadays are less willing than they were to care for their elderly relatives. Half the elderly in institutions were either single or married but childless, and others had only one child. In general, the children of the elderly continue to look after them if they can, and indeed there are far more old people continuously confined to bed in the homes of Britain than there are in all the "homes" and hospitals. The stereotype that critics of our social mores claim to be characteristic of today—the hard middle-aged woman who will not look after her old mother and is all too ready to dump her in a home so that she can continue to go to work to earn money towards buying the second car—is very largely a myth. The major causes of the increased demand for beds now are the larger numbers of elderly and the fewer children that these elderly people had, compared with their parents, when they were young. In the future the number of the old will continue to rise and soon they will be the parents of children born in the years of low birth rates, 1925–40.

Admission to a geriatric or psycho-geriatric unit is nowadays neither a life sentence nor a death sentence. Diagnosis, treatment and assessment can be both speedy and successful. In one well-known unit[2] the length of stay was reduced between 1947 and 1957 from

---

[1] Townsend, P. and Wedderburn, D., op. cit.
[2] Westropp, C., and Williams, M. *Health and Happiness in Old Age.* (Methuen. London 1960).

286 to 32 days. In psychiatric hospitals more than half of the elderly who are admitted have eminently treatable illnesses, and many of the others, though their dementia is incurable, improve enough in their behaviour to go home at least for a time. Others become fit enough for some different kind of care.

Gerontology

Any fundamental solution to the social and medical problems of ageing populations will have to await the fruits of research. Gerontology is a new branch of biology, a response to the skewing of the age curve, and it is rapidly expanding. But there is still no chair in the subject at any university in Britain. There is a vast amount to be learnt about the ageing process in cells, tissues, organs, and in species earlier than man. In time presumably we shall learn how to delay the course of ageing. But if the first practical outcome of this research is to lengthen life only after vigour has declined, which is the tendency at the moment, our difficulties will become worse. One hopes that in time means will be found of controlling and slowing down the ageing process so that degeneration is deferred.

Meanwhile, one partial remedy is within reach, but we have not grasped it firmly. The elderly 12% of our population contains many who continue to work; but others are forced into premature retirement by rigid rules. Several surveys of old people have brought to light a proportion who would like to continue to work but who, for reasons other than poor health, are unable to do so. To mobilise these people and continue to employ them involves decisions on social policy which are outside this book's scope except in one respect: forced retirement in those who are not ready is a fruitful cause of psychiatric disturbance—notably depressive illness—and one which is preventable.

Euthanasia

There is a further consequence of the ageing of the population. More people die in old age, often in extreme old age, and in many of them their bodies have survived their minds. Yet the advances of medical science, the discovery of antibiotics especially, and developments too in metallurgy and orthopaedic surgery, which have meant that the old can walk again within a short time of a fall that has fractured the neck of a femur, have given us the power to prolong such handicapped lives. Inevitably the nurses and doctors who look after them, and the relatives who, unrewarded by any glimmer of recognition from the senile, continue to visit them, must ask the question: is it worth it? Why not let them die? More often the question is not expressed but remains implicit. The remedy, too, is implicit and often enough unexpressed even by the doctor to himself. To withhold the last course of penicillin, to give enough tranquillising drugs to control noisiness and restlessness or enough barbiturate to produce sleep hardly qualify as euthanasia. After Nazi doctors carried out Hitler's order to wipe out the chronic sick, the mentally ill and the defective the word itself—like eugenics—has become soiled. It is reported[1] that in Germany 275,000 such were killed. Yet the problem remains —with its ethical, religious, social and criminal aspects—and from time to time becomes pressing. Controversy about euthanasia has doubtless been revived by current preoccupation with the problems of old age. But it is not exclusively so concerned. The question crops up, too, with grossly deformed new-born children bound to be severely subnormal, and not infrequently nowadays—such are the advances in medical science—in cases of prolonged coma. People who have suffered severe brain injuries either from haemorrhage or, particularly today, from motor accidents can be kept alive for months in respirators, fed through tubes, nursed with the greatest care, medicated to prevent pneumonia and yet with not the slightest chance of recovery to an independent existence. Who is to decide when to turn off the switch or withhold the drug?

A main part of the debate, which has raged on and off since the 1930s, has concerned the sufferer from incurable cancer. The questions that have been asked have been two. Has the patient in the full knowledge of his plight a right to ask for death? Has the doctor any right to carry out the patient's wishes, either deliberately or by leaving hypnotic or narcotic drugs in sufficient dosage within the patient's reach so that he can take them himself? One has the impression, after reading all the arguments so ably marshalled by Professor Glanville Williams[2] and by Mr St John Stevas,[3] arguments by moralists and Christians concerned with right and wrong and by lawyers concerned that the law should accord with reasonable practice, that things are probably best left as they are; that is to say, that the doctor will feel justified in giving sufficient amounts of a narcotic drug to relieve pain even if he knows that this will shorten the patient's life.

[1] Williams, G. *The Sanctity of Life and the Criminal Law.* (Faber and Faber. London, 1958).
[2] Williams, G. ibid.
[3] Stevas, N. St J. *Life, Death and the Law.* (Eyre and Spottiswoode. London, 1961).

The debate has in the main revolved round voluntary euthanasia, the right of someone with an incurable and painful disease, the pain of which cannot be properly relieved, to ask to be put to death. Certainly the safeguards suggested in the abortive English bill of 1936—a signed application by the applicant countersigned by two witnesses and forwarded with two medical certificates to an official referee who has personally to confirm that the patient understands the request—were formal to a gruesome degree, particularly as the lethal injection had then to be carried out in the presence of an official witness. Many of the frontiers between medicine, ethics and the law, such as the concept of criminal responsibility, are untidy. This is another. People must continue to trust their doctors to do what they think is right and in their best interests; doctors must continue to act as their consciences tell them and to assume that if they do they are very unlikely indeed to run foul of the law. Any written consent, even without the other paraphernalia—and at this stage of senile incomprehension or narcotic semi-stupor how many patients could give consent?—would make the mask of executioner too plain for most doctors to tolerate wearing it.

One further danger must be avoided. If the procedure is formalised doctors may well be both reluctant to embark on this course and more cautious about acting informally. There is a risk that more distraught relatives will take the law into their own hands. "Mercy killing" could increase.

Many of the advances of medicine in this age have left, as this book has shown, a legacy of ethical problems. They have been discussed as they have arisen. Who is to choose which among three suitable candidates should occupy a kidney machine? Whose pregnancy is to be terminated? Have the vices of experimental medicine and all the perplexing decisions in organ transplantation to remain unsettled? Resuscitation from cardiac arrest can be another occasion for the exercise of fine judgment, not least because an instant decision has to be taken by a nurse or a junior doctor; that is, unless some more senior doctor is prepared to say in advance that if such an event were to happen his patient is or is not to be resuscitated. Among all these momentous decisions, decisions of life and death, that have come upon medicine so fast and unexpectedly, those that concern euthanasia as described in this chapter are perhaps the least difficult to solve. Public debate is helpful, even if highly dramatised on television, but it will be a bad day for medicine if people cease to trust their doctors and if procedures are laid down replete with officials, referees, forms and committees. Given time the profession, as individuals rather than in any organised shape, will in all probability be able to work out some unofficial code, unwritten and unacknowledged, which in practice will assure the public that sensible, reasonable and just decisions are being taken. But time is needed, enough people have to experience the dilemma, adequate discussion within the profession at meetings and in journals has to flow before such an unofficial code can emerge to command majority assent. To hurry would be disastrous.

CHAPTER SEVEN

The Rise of Psychiatry

To describe the prodigious expansion of psychiatry, to isolate and analyse its causes, is to attempt something that transcends the bounds of medicine. Many of psychiatry's new characteristics arise admittedly from subjects discussed in earlier chapters. For instance it draws on statistical, experimental and other scientific methods. It makes use of drugs. It presents a new field, as does geriatrics, for preventive medicine. It has benefited handsomely from the attention no longer given to infectious disease. It is concerned with the increasing number of people now alive whose bodies have outlived their minds. Also, as with science, the stimulus of war has enormously speeded up its metamorphosis.

This chapter, therefore, is in a sense a culmination of what has gone before. But the changes and the causes of change go deeper than medicine however broadly defined, deep into the vast social upheavals and altered value systems of the twentieth century. The insight that Freud has given into the motives behind a person's behaviour; the expectations generated by economic security, a degree of social levelling, and improved health; the changed attitude to authority in all its forms; the decline in religious faith, replaced often enough today by materialist even by hedonistic values—all these have contributed in one way or another to the expansion of the conception of illness, a crucial feature of today's psychiatry. They have also aroused hopes—sometimes demands—that psychiatrists will provide solutions to problems that are really of social and philosophical concern. Psychiatrists are asked for cures for unhappiness and the misery of being an underdog, and for relief from accidie.

A doctor of fifty years ago would probably be as astonished by the lush growth of psychiatry as he would be by medicine's present control of infectious disease. For, as he formerly knew it, this was a branch of medicine practised by a handful of doctors in mental hospitals and regarded by most people in the profession as an odd and unrewarding backwater. Today it is vigorous and flourishing, rivalling general medicine and surgery in size. With its plans to set up a College of Psychiatrists it is claiming in Britain to have come of age and that for its further development it needs independent status within medicine.

Nor is this all. This doctor from the past would find that the transformation has brought psychiatry out from its isolated asylums into medicine. He would sense a changed attitude to mental disorders and neurosis both within the profession of medicine and among the general public. More surprising still, he would find psychiatrists working and welcome in spheres outside, or largely outside, medicine altogether; only an extraordinary extension of the meaning of the word illness could justify its use to describe the social problems that psychiatrists are increasingly called on to help with in the fields of education, marriage guidance, the rearing of children, employment, delinquency and criminal behaviour.

So far, in this book, the significant changes described in medicine have been broadly general, not very different perhaps in every advanced country. The expansion of psychiatry, however, springs from roots that are different in every country, roots going far back into each nation's history. The description that follows is of the trends in Britain. These are shared by many other countries, although the details may be different; they may indeed be becoming more universal for in the last thirty years or so Britain has, in many respects, been the pioneer.

War and the threat of war have often enough provided the stimulus for invention and technical advance in medicine. At the turn of the century, for example, Sir Almroth Wright was able to test and perfect his typhoid vaccine, which saved so many lives in later wars, on soldiers in the South African war. Again, the German search for synthetic antimalarial drugs to replace quinine in the 1920s, a search repeated in the United States twenty years later, has already been mentioned (page 51); and the large-scale manufacture of penicillin in the United States is unlikely to have been accomplished so quickly in peacetime.

Two world wars have undoubtedly played an important part in the metamorphosis of psychiatry in the last half-century, which has endowed its practitioners with a new authority and a bewildering variety of roles.

The Influence of Two Wars

Until 1930 or thereabouts the psychiatrist who worked in a mental hospital dealt very largely with the grosser degrees of psychosis. In such gross degree the term is equivalent to the legal word insanity and to the layman's word madness, and in order to be admitted to a mental hospital at all the patient had to be certified insane. The psychiatrist's experience, therefore, was confined to the organic psychoses such as can accompany damage to the brain by, for example, alcohol, syphilis, injury and senile degeneration, and to the severer forms of the two major non-organic psychoses, manic-depressive psychosis and schizophrenia. Other psychiatrists worked in institutions for mental defectives, caring for those with a severe degree of defect and also for those with milder degrees whose disturbed behaviour created a social problem. A few worked in private consulting practice, in private "homes" and hospitals or in the out-patient departments of some teaching hospitals and their experience was wider. It included the milder, non-"certifiable" degrees of the psychoses and, increasingly, the more severe degrees of neurosis or nervous illness. The remaining large division of the field of psychiatry, disorder of personality, which occupies today an appreciable part of a psychiatrist's time, was seldom seen unless the patient was in addition psychotic or neurotic.

The psychoses, which derive overwhelmingly either from brain disease, from general bodily disease, or from genetic (biochemical) causes, are little influenced by extraneous events in the world around. They are no more and no less common in wartime. On the other hand the neuroses, which are precipitated by stress and prevented by social solidarity, behave in a less predictable fashion. The cases of "shell-shock", which occurred so commonly in the appalling conditions of stress on the western front in the 1914–18 war, were at first thought, as the term implies, to be of organic origin. The condition was seen in the French army as early as August, 1914, and as the tempo of the war increased disturbing numbers of cases occurred in the British army too.

The organic label protected the sufferers from the accusations of moral weakness, brought by a patriotic public, that a diagnosis of neurosis would have entailed. It did not, however, deceive the alarmed administrators or the medical officers who had to treat an increasing number of these soldiers. The Battle of the Somme in 1916 produced several thousands of these casualties and this type of severe war neurosis remained a serious problem from then onwards. The records of the Ministry of Pensions show that, by 1939, 120,000 final or continuing pensions—the bulk of them, no doubt, originating in the war—had been awarded to sufferers from primary psychiatric disorders—15% of all pensioned disabilities.[1]

It seems that while the war continued there was a conspiracy to conceal the facts from the public. There was apprehension that any admission that large numbers of husbands, brothers and sons had developed neurotic illness would have a very harmful effect on morale; doctors and military authorities, sceptical and suspicious as usual and hard pressed by massive casualties, were convinced that frank acceptance of the facts would lead to an epidemic of invalidism and evasion of duty; there was the familiar difficulty of distinguishing neurosis from malingering; only the officers in action themselves favoured the removal from duty of those who showed these symptoms —naturally, as their own lives might well depend upon these sick or, at the least, unreliable companions.

The silence did not long outlast the war, and as a result of the questions he asked on the subject in the House of Lords in 1920 Lord Southborough was made the chairman of a committee of enquiry. The report on shell-shock was issued in 1922.[2] Even at this distance it is seen to be a most enlightened document, and its recommendations on measures to prevent war neurosis are still valid—selection, training, observation for signs of stress, avoidance of excessive fatigue, periods of rest and convalescence. It states: "As a result [of faulty methods of recruitment] a great number of men who were ill-suited to stand the strain of military service, whether by temperament or their past or present condition of mental and nervous health, were admitted into the army; there is no doubt that such men contributed a very high proportion of the cases of hysteria and traumatic neurosis commonly called 'shell-shock'."

These conclusions had been largely anticipated five years earlier by the Americans. Alarmed by the reports of "shell-shock" in the British army they had sent Dr T. W. Salmon to England in 1917 to make enquiries. His report, which was largely responsible for the introduction of selection and of psychiatrists to the American military scene, predicted that the "wide prevalence of neurosis among soldiers will direct attention to the fact that this kind of illness has been almost wholly ignored". He called for a revision of the medical and the popular attitude towards functional nervous diseases.[3]

The experiences of the 1914–18 war left many thousands of men under treatment for neurosis. Hundreds of doctors in the army

[1] Ahrenfeldt, R. H., *Psychiatry in the British Army in the Second World War*. (Routledge and Kegan Paul. London, 1958).
[2] *Report of the War Office Committee of Enquiry into "Shell-Shock"*. (H.M.S.O. London, 1922).
[3] Ahrenfeldt, R. H., op. cit.

gained experience in recognising and trying to treat these illnesses and on their return to civil life recognised their prevalence in the population in peacetime. The public began to be aware of a shadowy land between the poles of organic illness and moral weakness. As a result, at least a start was made in providing medical aid for this hitherto unrecognised legion of patients even if, for many reasons, the subsequent advance was at a snail's pace.

Out-patient clinics were gradually established in teaching hospitals and at other university centres and a handful of specialised clinics and hospitals were opened, notably the Tavistock Clinic in 1920. The Maudsley Hospital, built in 1915, was used as a war hospital and later by the Ministry of Pensions for cases of "shell-shock". In 1923 it reverted to its original purpose as a hospital where early cases of mental illness could be admitted—voluntarily, instead of having to be certified insane—and its out-patient service began.

The Royal Commission on Lunacy and Mental Disorder of 1924, besides making, in its report, the revolutionary suggestion that patients should be allowed to seek treatment voluntarily in all mental hospitals, proposed that local authorities should be encouraged to establish out-patient clinics. Except for children they never did, at least in any appreciable numbers.

Progress was tantalisingly slow. Most of England's psychiatrists, like their patients, were locked up behind the walls and gates of mental hospitals. In general the medical profession was hostile, and even as late as 1946 Dr C. P. Blacker was still reporting widespread prejudice against psychiatry and a failure on the part of many, but not all, general practitioners to appreciate the prevalence and the nature of the neuroses. The stigma of mental illness, which ensured that a patient with a psychosis only went to a mental hospital as a last resort, still largely marked the neuroses too. These much commoner illnesses, in spite of the slow change in public attitude and the reluctant provision of some facilities for treating them, continued to be concealed under names—effort syndrome, disordered action of the heart, anaemia, atypical migraine, dyspepsia—that implied an organic rather than an emotional origin. Such a "diagnosis" spared the sufferer from having to bear voiced or implied accusations of moral weakness as well as his symptoms. "Snap out of it", "pull yourself together" continued to be the medical as well as the lay advice given to a neurotic patient, who had to bite back the obvious retort—"I would if I could." All too often such patients were referred to any department other than the psychiatric department of a hospital and remained untreated, despised and ill-understood.

I

Nevertheless by the beginning of the Second World War psychiatry had made some impressive strides, and the role of emotional stress in causing neurotic illness was far better understood. In fact a committee of eighteen eminent psychiatrists suggested in 1938 that as a result of air-raids on cities psychiatric casualties might outnumber physical casualties by as much as three to one. They expected an epidemic of psychiatric illness involving perhaps three or four million people in Britain and suggested that a massive organisation would have to be created to cope with them. The Government took this advice seriously, although preparations were made on nothing like this scale.[1] Partly perhaps because a year of war passed before heavy bombing raids began these casualties never materialised. More probably the reason was that the protection that high group morale confers against neurotic illness had been much underestimated. In the event, instead of an epidemic of panic, hysteria and neurotic reactions there was a bathetic but nevertheless unpleasant epidemic of bedwetting among children evacuated from their homes. This may have been due in part to anxiety caused by separation from parents, but in the main it was an unmasking of one of the more sordid aspects of urban life at that time.[2]

This astonishing and topsy-turvy confounding of expert opinion underlines both the public's ignorance of social conditions in its midst and the psychiatrists' ignorance then of factors influencing morale and group-behaviour. In the last twenty years each field has been much more intensively studied and both form part of the territory of social psychiatry. A great deal has been learnt of the preventive and therapeutic influence of groups. This has become one of the most flourishing growing points of the specialty, and one, moreover, in which psychiatry has significantly escaped from the strict confines of medicine and invaded the broader field of sociology.

In the Second World War, although psychiatrists were not called upon to treat vast numbers of civilian casualties they had many other roles to play. At the beginning the same mistakes were made as had encumbered the hospitals twenty-five years before. The War Office ignored the recommendations of their own "shell-shock" report and rejected in 1939 any preselection procedure aimed at excluding those likely to become psychiatric casualties. Selection, once a man was in the army, was opposed on the ground that it was unfair to deprive any man of his right to become a field marshal if he could, and pre-

[1] Titmuss, R. M. *History of the Second World War: problems of social policy.* (H.M.S.O. London, 1950.)
[2] *Our Towns: a close-up.* A study for the Women's Group on Public Welfare. (Oxford University Press. London, 1943.)

selection was opposed because of the inability or unwillingness of recruiting boards to distinguish neurosis from malingering. There was the same hostility to psychiatric ideas and methods from the medical profession[1] and from the army administration. The latter, concerned to produce manpower from a limited pool, opposed any system of selection as it robbed them of men. It would have been more far-sighted to fit limited men into jobs to suit their limited capacities so that Britain's scanty manpower could have been used to the best advantage.

Gradually the facts of the situation forced changes to be made. Breakdown rates of those so hastily recruited soon became alarming and many men had to be discharged. Techniques of personnel-selection derived from industrial psychology were evolved and, instead of being discharged, some handicapped men were transferred to protected employment. By the end of the war techniques of job analysis and of selection, pioneered by psychiatrists (a psychiatrist has had a medical training; most psychologists have not), had become universally accepted because they were efficient. Nevertheless, discharge rates continued to be high and in 1943 psychiatric disorders caused one-third of all medical discharges from the army.

Selection of officers soon became a concern of the growing number of army psychiatrists. The bankruptcy of orthodox selection—"I know a good man when I see him"—very soon became painfully clear. Both the rejection-rate at officers' training units and the breakdown-rate in officers were high. Psychiatrists evolved techniques using an intelligence test, an interview and a questionnaire which soon proved as valuable as a five-week period of observation by a skilled commanding officer. Later the War Office Selection Boards used W. R. Bion's leaderless-group technique as an aid in officer-selection—a highly original and very successful means of bringing out the personal qualities of members of a small group required to perform a set task. This device has been adopted by the Civil Service as one of their methods of selecting recruits. Of late, out of the applicants for entry to the hundred or so places in the Administrative class about 600 choose to be examined by this method (method II).

In general, since the war, the reasoning underlying selection for jobs, and the techniques developed during the war, have permeated industry. The principle of trying to select the man for the job rather than of relying on trial and error is spreading, and training courses are now commonplace. Naturally when jobs are plentiful and people

[1] Rees, J. R. *The Shaping of Psychiatry by War.* (Norton. New York, 1945).

to fill them are scarce the policy cannot get very far even if the principle is granted.

To return to the theme: in the Second World War preselection, selection and rejection, as in the earlier war, were most popular nearest to the fighting. They were popular with the regimental doctor and the commanding officers for obvious reasons. Further back they aroused intense hostility. Outspoken criticism came from the very top—"I am sure it would be sensible to restrict as much as possible the work of these gentlemen, who are capable of doing an immense amount of harm."[1] But his doctor did not on this occasion agree with him. In the preface to his book, *The Anatomy of Courage*, Lord Moran[2] states ". . . if an Army is being prepared to fight it ought to begin by eliminating those who are incapable of fighting." Later on, and excluding from his discussion those who have undergone exceptional and prolonged stress, he continues: "there is no sense in holding on to men without stability who are blown over by the first breath of battle."

Other nations at the same time were adopting exactly the same attitude. The Americans had a much more efficient selection-rejection procedure, which included a psychiatrist on the selection board, and they have always rejected for service a far higher proportion of recruits than the British. The United States attitude is well expressed in the words: "The Army is an organisation for the defence of the nation and is not to be considered a corrective institution." A colonel in the Red Army is reported to have said[3] of dullards: "There is no place for any dull men in the modern army; we keep them out, or if they get in, we send them back to industry at once."

The malign influence of the psychiatrist on morale is of course a matter of opinion and hardly open to proof or disproof. Official army statistics of desertion are, however, interesting. The death sentence for cowardice was abolished in 1930. In the 1914–18 war 3,080 men were sentenced to death for cowardice and desertion and 346 were executed. Despite this deterrent the desertion rate in that war was 10·26 per 1,000 strength per year. In the 1939–45 war the corresponding figure was 6·89. Conditions, certainly, were very different in the two wars with, in the later one, many "combatants" in less danger than their relatives at home. None the less, the figures

---

[1] Churchill, W. S. *The Second World War.* vol. 4. appendix C. (Cassell. London, 1951).
[2] Moran, Lord. *The Anatomy of Courage.* (Constable. London, 1945).
[3] Rees, J. R., op. cit.

do not support the charge of morale-sapping and incidentally will be of interest to the opponents of the death penalty for the crimes of civil life.

At the beginning of the last war the army employed eight doctors with psychiatric experience; by the end there were 300. Naturally, as well as pioneering methods of selection, these doctors were intimately concerned with the diagnosis and treatment of battle casualties—and developed new techniques like abreaction with barbiturates and amphetamine in the process. These techniques continue to be used in the treatment of some cases of neurosis in peacetime. They are components in the psychiatrists' new found armoury of physical methods of treatment. The experiments in the selection of officers, studies of the factors underlying morale, and success in the treatment of returned prisoners of war underlined the immense importance of social and group factors in influencing peoples' thinking, feeling and behaviour. Questions of identity, of role, of belonging, of communication, of attitudes to authority were shown to be powerful determinants of behaviour and capable both of causing symptoms and of becoming therapeutic.

The Study of Social Setting

The systematic study of group-dynamics belongs more to sociology than to medicine, but the fillip that it received from army psychiatry provided a momentum which it never had before. Human relations in industry, personnel-management, industrial unrest, the study of leadership, hierarchies, the management of prisons—these are all topics that have sprung into prominence since the war. In the sphere of medicine at present there is a growing interest in communications within general hospitals. The word is used in a special sense, like so many words in the social sciences, and does not mean, though it includes, the efficiency of telephone systems and portering. In the current context it deals with relationships between patients and various grades of staff and more particularly between the various groups and grades of staff themselves. To take some simple examples: when nurses can talk to the Sister and be taken notice of, and when they can be sure that any notes that they write will be read and remembered by the ward doctor, the patients may recover more quickly; when resident nurses and doctors can have regular meetings with the catering staff, that chronic disgruntlement and grousing, which is so characteristic of institutional life and which hampers efficiency, melts away. The doctors, less lordly and laggard than usual, are beginning to show enthusiasm for these new ideas, and they are penetrating even to the staffs of the teaching hospitals, thanks mainly to the Ministry of Health and to the two voluntary organisations that give encouragement and funds, King Edward's Hospital Fund for London and the Nuffield Provincial Hospitals Trust.

In psychiatric hospitals themselves the success of whatever treatments have at one time or another been available has been heavily influenced by the setting in which they are given. Even in the eighteenth century exceptional people like Pinel in Paris and the Tukes at York and, in the nineteenth, Gardiner Hill, Pritchard and Conolly had shown that the phenomena of mental illness varied with the conditions in which patients were looked after. Good administration, an atmosphere of non-restraint, trust, the preservation of personal identity, and the encouragement of useful occupation were time and again shown to be therapeutic, but these principles seldom outlasted the reign of the innovator and then the old regime of harshness, idleness, squalor and padlocks re-established itself.

Since the last war the effect of the milieu in which mentally ill people are treated has been exhaustively studied and analysed. Concepts of a "therapeutic community" and of "administrative therapy" have been established and these ideas put into practice. A WHO report[1] has listed the requirements as including preservation of a patient's individuality; the assumption that patients are trustworthy and should be given responsibility; full occupation for all patients; and a system of rewards for good behaviour. "Therapeutic communities" are as various as the authors who write about them, but they all enshrine at least these principles and many go much farther, particularly those that attempt to treat neurotic patients and to remould disordered personalities. In them, according to a recent exposition,[2] the following principles must hold: they should be small enough for everybody to know everyone else; meetings should be held regularly and all the people in the community attend, patients, doctors and other staff; at these meetings the underlying philosophy is psychodynamic and all subjects including the motives and behaviour of others are freely discussed; the authority of hierarchical figures, doctors and nurses, is diminished and both they and the patients are encouraged to examine their roles and the psychological meaning of day-to-day events within the community; "communication" is free; the aim is to encourage everybody to understand

[1] WHO. *Expert Committee on Mental Health.* 3rd report. (Geneva, 1953).
[2] Clark, D. H. (1965). *Brit. J. Psychiat.* **111**, 947.

their roles, their attitudes, their motives and behaviour in this social context. Most neurosis units, many day hospitals and some mental hospitals, or parts of them, are nowadays run in accordance with these principles. Limited use is made of them, too, in out-patient psychiatric practice.

The lessons that have been learnt about the harmful effects of some institutions and the "therapeutic" characteristics of others have an obvious place in penal reform. Both in Britain and elsewhere very tentative efforts are being made in the prison service to apply some of the principles—smallness, non-restraint, full occupation, a diminution in the aloofness of hierarchical figures—especially in Borstals. According to one authority:[1] "Borstal staffs learned early that authoritarianism increases the distance between staff and prisoner, and that this makes it much more difficult either to understand or to influence him," and the diffusion of staff with experience of Borstal methods throughout the prison service had led to a more general change in the attitude of staff towards the prisoners. The "Norwich experiment", begun in 1958, in which it was planned that each staff member in prisons would personally interest himself in twenty prisoners, has been superseded by "group counselling". This counselling, soon in operation in a score of prisons and Borstals, involves one prison officer in group discussions with eight prisoners. The topics brought up include family relationships, fears, discipline and discharge problems.[2]

In comparison with group methods used in psychiatry changes like these are in their infancy and there are, as yet, no opinions about their effect on behaviour after the prisoner has been released. All agree, however, that they have achieved a lessening of tension within the prison. Critics[3] say that these methods affect only 1,000 of the 30,000 prisoners in England and Wales, that liberal experiments are often ephemeral and are given undue prominence in official reports and in the press, and that policy is facing two ways because "90% of the effective activity of authority in prisons is unconstructive or actually damaging". One should not underestimate the difficulties. The pioneers of the therapeutic community movement in mental hospitals needed great courage to prod and persuade their staffs to relinquish the keys, the manner and other trappings of their authority, to trust patients and to risk the anger of the community as a consequence of failure. Much has been achieved in open prisons and

[1] Rose, G. *The Struggle for Penal Reform.* (Stevens. London, 1961).
[2] Rolph, C. H. *Commonsense about Crime and Punishment.* (Gollancz. London, 1961).
[3] Sington, D., and Playfair, G. *Crime, Punishment and Cure.* (Secker and Warburg. London, 1965).

in Borstals. To go farther reformers must perforce encounter more opposition from a community still convinced of the virtues of the punitive and deterrent aspects of imprisonment and will have to contend with the wariness of prisoners. Of these, many either have a long ingrained allegiance to a delinquent subculture, or have as a distinguishing characteristic an incapacity to develop group feelings at all.

But it is a long step from trying to mitigate the harmful effects of institutions to regarding prisoners as patients in need of treatment—group treatment—to cure their antisocial behaviour. Before this step is taken, if it ever is, social psychiatrists would have to produce evidence that their methods work and are more effective than present penal methods or the passage of time alone; society would have to reorientate itself to confront the criminal rather than his "symptom", the crime, so that, if necessary, a trivial offence might entail a life-time of "treatment". The time has come when psychiatry, apart from treating sick individuals wherever they are, in industry, in prisons, in schools and universities, may turn its attention to the functioning of these groups themselves. It has already looked fruit-fully at its own institutions; it is looking at industry and at penal establishments. There are those who would go farther. Schools and colleges, armies, child care, international relations, according to these enthusiasts, are all institutional fields which the concepts of social psychiatry can illuminate.

It would be inaccurate to claim that all these developments—selection, industrial psychiatry, job analysis, group therapy and the physiology of institutions—derived solely from the work of psychia-trists in the army. They had other sources in many cases, but the pressing needs of war provided the stimulus for adaptation, ingenuity and fresh ideas. It is ironical that Dr J. R. Rees and his team, so many of them raised under the influence of Freud's genius, should have been pioneers in social psychiatry. Psychoanalysis is the paradigm of individual treatment. Their distinction has been to apply what he found out about man's mental functioning to man as a member of a group larger than his immediate family.

Other psychiatrists in the army and the other services were employed in treating casualties, those who had never seen any fighting as well as those who had. In all, in the five years from September, 1939, to June, 1944, 118,000 men and women[1] were

[1] *Report on the Work of Psychologists and Psychiatrists in the Services.* (H.M.S.O. London, 1947).

discharged from the British armed forces for psychiatric reasons. It was perhaps this steady march of undramatic neurotic illness—for the dramatic hysterical comas, amnesias and paralyses of the First World War were seldom seen—which brought home to the medical profession, and later to the public, the prevalence of psychiatric disorders.

In addition, these 300–400 service psychiatrists, many of them hitherto locked up in mental hospitals with their patients, mixed with ordinary people and other doctors in officers' messes. They must have been good ambassadors.

After the war and with the coming of the national health service the demand for specialist psychiatric services for neurotic patients became insistent and the facilities were gradually expanded. In the past twenty years in Britain out-patient clinics, formerly concentrated in the voluntary hospitals, have been opened in virtually every general hospital of any size. In the years 1946–65 the number of clinics increased from 216 to over 600. The number of out-patients seen (see Table 6) increases year by year, but the demand for consultations seems never to be satisfied and waiting lists are commonly long.

TABLE 6

England and Wales

	Total Psychiatric Out-Patients (thousands)	New Psychiatric Out-Patients (thousands)
1950	466	97
1952	568	108
1954	772	132
1956	895	143
1958	1,021	152
1960	1,265	167
1962	1,383	185
1964	1,433	197
1966	1,460	212

These figures include child guidance and subnormality.
Source: Ministry of Health Annual Reports.

The Influence of Freud

Over a period of forty-six years this revolutionary explorer of the human mind published a body of books, papers, essays, lectures and case-studies containing $3\frac{1}{2}$ million words.[1] His contributions to human knowledge have probably been as great as those of anyone in the twentieth century, though some people, behaviourists and others, would vigorously dispute this. His work is of peculiar significance because man's increasing ability to control his environment has now focused attention on his urgent necessity to control himself. It is at first sight paradoxical that Freud's greatest achievement should have been in the realms of normal psychology and philosophy rather than therapy, for he generalised with great freedom from studying only himself and a handful of sick people. But this is not really surprising: in the medical sciences a study of diseased people, of pathology, has often before shed clear light on normal function. Freud produced the first comprehensive dynamic theory of personality, and it has been suggested that his success was in fact largely due to his working with patients and to his being a doctor, for "only miserably sick people in need of help can be encouraged to abandon their defences one by one and eventually reveal their innermost secrets".[2] His success can be judged by the extent to which his concepts have permeated the language of ordinary people and the literature and drama of Western culture. He and his colleagues and their translators have produced a number of new words, and new meanings of old words, that are now part of the English language, though often enough they are inaccurately used: the unconscious, repression, resistance, abreaction, superego, transference, regression, libido, id, wish-fulfilment—these are just a few.

It has been most unfortunate that the word psychoanalysis has acquired so many meanings. It means first the body of theory that Freud established; secondly, it defines a research weapon, mainly based on free association, which he developed; thirdly, it is a technique of treatment based again on free association, the interpretation of dreams and on "the transference" (the patient's emotional attachment to the doctor) which he used in helping neurotic patients; lastly it is used to describe the organisation of those who employ these techniques, closed to those who are not steeped in the literature of the subject and who have not had a personal analysis.

Freud's distinctive contributions have been to demonstrate the importance to all of us of mental processes of which we are unaware and to show that experiences and relationships in early life are of cardinal importance in the development of personality. His influence

[1] Stafford-Clark, D. *What Freud Really Said*. (Macdonald. London, 1965).
[2] Murray, H. A. and Kluckhohn, C. in *Personality in Nature, Culture and Psychiatry*. (Jonathan Cape. London, 1953).

looms large over our changed attitude to the rearing of children, to education, to the roles of parents, and to sexual and other relationships.

In medicine itself the effects of his theories, his discoveries and language have been complex, slowly pervasive and tortuous rather than direct. In Britain his direct followers have never been numerous, and psychoanalysis, the movement, has never wielded a great deal of power in psychiatry or in medicine. In the United States, on the other hand, ever since Freud delivered his Five Lectures on Psychoanalysis there in 1909 his influence on the development of psychiatry has been formidable. Only there was it considered prudent, if a bright young man wanted the best training for a lifetime in psychiatry, for him to embark on a personal analysis.

Elsewhere the hostility and ridicule which Freudian ideas originally aroused in the medical profession and elsewhere slowly abated in the years between the wars. Neurotic symptoms began to be taken more seriously. There was pressure from literary sources; there was pressure from patients who felt that hope at last had dawned for those with neurotic symptoms who had for so long been ignored by their doctors; and there was pressure from a handful of enthusiasts within the profession. Gradually, particularly among younger doctors, it became plain that to dismiss, as "functional", a patient whose symptoms on investigation turned out to have no physical basis, and to do no more about it, was inadequate. The illness deserved, and increasingly got, more enquiry, sympathetic listening, an effort to uncover emotional and social factors behind it; and if necessary the patient was referred as an out-patient for psychiatric help. The psychiatrists, then as now, were seldom psychoanalysts, but they mostly had a dynamic approach and had been influenced by Freud as by McDougall, William James, Janet, Adolf Meyer, Jung, Ross, Adler and Ryle. Their psychotherapy was seldom psychoanalysis, but it made use of an assortment of techniques aiming at various degrees of "depth" to suit each patient and his illness. Some help at least could be given. Not the least of Freud's claims to fame has been his establishment of a beachhead. In his struggles to help patients with neurotic illnesses the modern doctor starts from here, even if he goes off in an entirely different direction, to explore for example the field of social psychiatry or of treatment with the new psychotropic drugs. Many criticisms can be made of details of the body of psychoanalytical theory, of its excesses, its omissions, and of the failure of its supporters to produce any scientific evidence of its effectiveness as a technique of therapy; but it cannot be denied that

Freud's influence was one of the most potent causes of psychiatry's growth in this century.

The Success of Physical Treatment and Drugs

Only a few kinds of neurosis are regarded as suitable for psychoanalysis or any other form of analytical psychotherapy. Apart from the type of neurosis, lack of intelligence, time and money and the necessity of earning a living severely limit the number of people who can benefit from psychoanalysis. Even so, psychoanalysts and other psychotherapists have been remarkably shy of collecting or publishing their results. The Berlin Psychoanalytic Institute in the years 1920–30 accepted 312 patients for psychoanalysis: 112 dropped out for one reason or another; and 91% of the remainder, which was only 58% of the original number, improved or recovered.[1] Other psychotherapists report figures showing usually that 60–70% of their patients recover or are much improved by the end of treatment. Professor Eysenck[2] quotes the "spontaneous" recovery rates in two groups of American neurotic patients treated without psychotherapy in any formal sense of the word as "about two-thirds". More recently[3] he has written: "as is well known, the rate of spontaneous remission in severe neurotic disorders is such that some 45 percent recover after one year and over 70 percent after two years, without any form of psychiatric treatment."

No doubt there are difficulties in defining exactly what is meant by "recovery" or "much improvement" in the psychoneuroses. That there can still be doubt after all this time about the efficacy of psychoanalysis and psychotherapy in comparison with the effect of no treatment or of being a name on a waiting list is disturbing. Have all those millions of hours of careful and expensive listening been a waste of time? Do those patients who get better do so because the passage of time allows their illnesses to remit or because of some virtue in the treatment? Only more time and large-scale controlled studies comparing the results of psychotherapy with that of other forms of treatment, and with no treatment at all, can give the answer.

There can be no such doubts about the success of some forms of physical treatment for the psychoses. Freud himself freely admitted that, apart from throwing some light on some of the mental mechanisms that psychotic patients display, psychoanalysis could contribute

[1] Freud, S. *New Introductory Lectures on Psychoanalysis*. (Hogarth Press and Institute of Psychoanalysis. London, 1936).
[2] Eysenck, H. J. *Uses and Abuses of Psychology*. (Penguin Books. London, 1953).
[3] Eysenck, H. J. *Fact and Fiction in Psychology*. (Penguin Books. London, 1965).

nothing towards an understanding of the reasons why these illnesses crop up, or towards the treatment of them. The organic psychoses— associated with degenerative changes in the brain, with infections, injuries and intoxications—have obvious causes and their treatment is only possible if the underlying cause can be removed. The more mysterious non-organic psychoses, mainly schizophrenia (including the paranoid varieties that can arise in middle life or later) and manic depressive psychosis, account for two-thirds of the admissions to mental hospitals and for a great deal of illness in the community outside. Both have a strong bent to run in families and both have a tendency to spontaneous remission far stronger in the case of mania and depression than of schizophrenia. There is also a liability to a relapse later on. Schizophrenia, but not the manic-depressive psychosis, tends strongly to become chronic so that more than half the patients with this illness used to remain in hospital, once they had been admitted, for the rest of their lives.

Until the middle of the 1930s psychiatrists could only stand and watch the natural course of these diseases. They could do little or nothing to alter it. For more than thirty years, beginning with Sakel's deep insulin treatment in 1933, and von Meduna's convulsion therapy introduced as far back as 1928, one physical treatment for these diseases has followed another. Many, like the original two, have been abandoned: deep insulin, as already mentioned, because even after twenty years' use there was no scientific proof that it really improved the illness;[1] chemical convulsion treatment because, for both patient and doctor, it was too barbarous to survive. But many have survived, notably electric convulsion treatment (ECT), various forms of brain surgery for occasional use, and a range of effective drugs. The drugs include the versatile phenothiazine group, and the imipramine series of antidepressants (Tofranil, Tryptizol, Aventyl etc.). The latter have already been conclusively shown[2] to be effective in certain depressive illnesses; the former, especially in the shape of the original member of the group, chlor- promazine (Largactil), have been responsible for a continuing spate of papers in the past twelve years. Phenothiazines can control dis- turbed and aggressive behaviour due to any cause and many people believe that they can cure schizophrenia or at least permanently suppress its symptoms. Neither group of drugs is by any means perfect, and perhaps a quarter of apparently suitable people fail to

---

[1] Ackner, B., Harris, A. and Oldham, A. J. (1957), *Lancet*, **i,** 607.
[2] "Clinical Trial of the Treatment of Depressive Illness". (*M.R.C.* report). 1965, *Brit. Med. J.*, **i,** 881.

respond to them; but their success means that there is hope that before long drugs will be found that will more certainly correct the biochemical abnormality that must be the core of these psychoses.

To say that the other theories of the origin of schizophrenia do not really hold water would be dogmatic and unappreciative of fresh ideas. Psychodynamic theories are, however, very unconvincing, and this is as true of older theories as it is of the new ideas of Lidz and Bateson and of the existentialist views of Laing.[1] These concentrate upon the "schizophrenogenic" family and in particular on the ambiguous attitude of the mother in these families. Mothers of schizophrenic patients are often indeed odd, cold but narrowly passionate, and inconsistent, and they manage to combine intense concern over detail with emotional rejection. But it is at least as plausible to postulate that both the patient's illness and the mother's peculiarity arise from genetic factors as to suppose that the one causes the other. The social theories of aetiology are even more unsatisfactory and derive from epidemiological studies and from the selective preponderance of this disease in social classes IV and V and in the socially disintegrated centres of large cities. They gain a little support from the convincing demonstration in recent years that the established illness is responsive to changes in social surroundings, but to regard these factors as crucial rather than as merely contributing raises more questions than it answers. Social factors and the family may well have a very important influence in causing a relapse of the treated case and it is important that research into these aspects of this baffling disease should continue.

In parenthesis one should perhaps remember that there is no logical reason why failure of a line of therapy based on a particular theory of causation should damn the theory itself. Freudian or Laingian theory *might* be correct even though their methods of therapy failed to benefit schizophrenics. Furthermore, both genetic-biochemical theory and Freudian theory could be correct. They are not necessarily incompatible as they operate at different levels and employ different categories of concepts.

It is fruitless to argue whether ECT and these new drugs or the administrative changes already discussed have contributed more to the quite extraordinary changes that mental hospitals have undergone in the last fifteen years—as startling as any in medicine. They have been synergistic—each has helped the other. In some cases improvement following administrative changes preceded the introduction of the drugs; in others the effects of drug treatment facilitated the

[1] Laing, R. D. *The Divided Self.* (Tavistock Publications. London, 1960).

opening of doors, full occupation, encouragement of initiative, freer communication and the restoration of an atmosphere of hope. Certainly, the physical treatments encourage the hope that this time, as has never happened before in institutional psychiatry, there will be no relapse, after individual enthusiasm wanes, into an atmosphere of repression and neglect.

The consequences have been far-reaching. Within mental hospitals disturbed behaviour has melted away as a problem and become quite exceptional. The length of time needed to treat a psychotic illness has shortened: in the case of a severe attack of depression from six months to seven weeks; in the case of a first attack of schizophrenia from ten months to eight weeks. The improved atmosphere, the prospects of a brisk cure, and the provisions of the enlightened Mental Health Act of 1959, which came into force late in 1960, have between them led to an increased demand for treatment in hospital, shown in the steady rise in admissions from 59,000 in 1951 to 114,000 in 1960. In 1967 they were 169,000; but 1960 is the last year for which figures can be properly compared with admissions before the Act. At any one time perhaps only 5% of the patients in hospitals are there under any kind of compulsion; indeed, the difficulty nowadays may be not to persuade the patient to enter hospital but to persuade him to leave when he is well enough to do so. In spite of an increased demand for treatment, and the rise in the number of patients admitted, there has been a fall in the total number of patients in hospital in the past ten years. Whether, as forecast, this fall will continue is uncertain. Indeed some hospitals which led the field are now finding that their numbers are stationary or even beginning to increase again. Some figures illustrating these trends are shown in Chart IV on the next page.

One of the reasons for the increase in the number of admissions is that schizophrenia has been converted from an untreatable to a partially treatable illness. Some patients, as has always happened, have a single attack from which they recover and are never seen in hospital again. There may today be more of these. Others who formerly would have remained in hospital for the rest of their lives now recover but remain liable to further attacks, or only improve and have to be readmitted on many occasions subsequently for further treatment. A few ultimately have to remain permanently in hospital. The pessimistic view is that the only effect of treatment is to delay by some years the inevitable progress of these patients to ultimate chronic invalidism. But this is not the view of most psychiatrists. Most of them have patients under their care who are drug-dependent, as are patients with diabetes or pernicious anaemia. So long as they take their medication they remain well and at work; if for some reason—incomplete insight into the need, prejudice against taking drugs, unpleasant side-effects, discouragement from relatives —they stop, a relapse is inevitable, and readmission is needed, in a few weeks or months. Two studies[1][2] have shown that probably between a quarter and a half of the schizophrenic patients out of hospital may not be taking their drugs or not be taking them regularly or in the correct dose. This problem is not, by the way, confined to psychiatric patients but is characteristic of tuberculous outpatients as well, and perhaps, too, of those having drugs to control high blood pressure.

Numbers and admissions to hospitals for mental illness   Chart IV

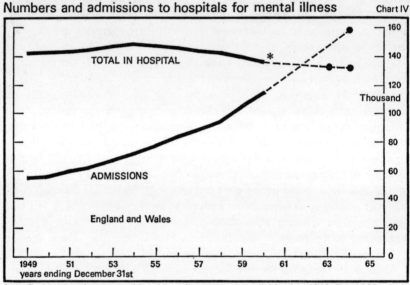

* No figures exactly comparable with earlier years are available after 1960. The 1963 figure derived from "A Census of Patients in Psychiatric Beds" 1963 by Eileen M. Brooke, H.M.S.O. London. The other later estimates have been supplied by Mr. G. D. Tidey of the Ministry of Health.

Source: Registrar General's Statistical Reviews 1952-53 and 1960. Supplements on Mental Health.

The ease and speed with which many psychotic illnesses can be treated today and the rarity of seriously disturbed behaviour have encouraged a new trend. Properly designed psychiatric units in general hospitals are now regarded as the ideal place in which to treat the bulk of psychotic illness. Many seriously ill patients, too,

[1] Parkes, G. M., Brown, G. W. and Monck, E. M. (1962), *Brit. Med. J.*, **i,** 972.
[2] Willcox, D. R. C., Gillan, R. U. and Hare, E. H. (1965), *Brit. Med. J.*, **ii,** 790.

particularly those with depressive illnesses, can be successfully treated in day hospitals, and some even as out-patients attending general hospital clinics. But herein lies a danger: that if the bulk of acute psychiatry is dealt with outside mental hospitals these will again become neglected, difficult to staff, and filled with patients for whom hope has been abandoned.

The Trend to Community Care

The treatment of patients in or near their homes, and the special problem of the incompletely recovered schizophrenic patient, have made the provision of preventive, supportive and aftercare measures, loosely summarised as "community care", more than ever necessary. Hostels, day centres, occupation centres, sheltered workshops, home visiting, social clubs are some of the facilities being provided now for the mentally ill as they have for decades been provided by local health authorities for the mentally subnormal. The general practitioner and the hospital doctor are naturally involved too in this preventive work and, in this field at least, the rigid barriers between the three branches of Britain's health service are collapsing.

The era of "community care" which we have entered now should be contrasted with two earlier phases. Until the middle of the nineteenth century the vast majority of the mentally ill existed outside mental hospitals. They were either at home—and in the overcrowded squalid conditions of the towns of the industrial revolution were often in great distress—or in prisons or workhouses or in private madhouses, which were entirely unsupervised and were run for profit. In 1850 only 7,000 people of the 19 million population of England and Wales were in public asylums.[1] This was the era of "community neglect", which Shaftesbury's humane exertions were meant to end. The system he wished to substitute, of small institutions properly run, of inspection, and of safeguarded certification, was distorted in the course of the next few decades. Instead, vast and soulless asylums, some with as many as 3,000 beds, were built and were impossible to run humanely. Only the severely ill could ever get into them because of the rigid regulation of certification and, once they were there, the effect of the institution itself was such that they seldom came out.

Thus by 1914, of a total of 36 million people, 138,000 were in mental hospitals, homes and so on. This was the era of "community

[1] Jones, Kathleen. *Mental Health and Social Policy, 1845–1959.* (Routledge and Kegan Paul. London, 1960).

K

rejection", from which we are just emerging. If the wheel is not to turn full circle money and resources will have to be devoted to "community care" on a larger scale than at present. More psychiatrists, more social workers and more buildings will be needed and more effort from general practitioners.

The ripples of the success of psychopharmacology have spread farther still. Psychotic illness has lost some of its dread with the prospect of such effective help at hand. There is no longer a conspiracy of silence about the subject and it, in common with other psychiatric topics, has become a frequent subject of articles in the press and of programmes on the radio and television. People visit their doctors earlier in their illnesses instead of as a last resort.

The initial stages of these illnesses are, however, the most difficult in which to establish a diagnosis—and an accurate diagnosis is very important. The distinction is not easy even for a specialist between a mild endogenous depression with some anxiety symptoms and a neurotic anxiety state with some depression (precipitated in a rather unstable person by some stress in his environment)—such is the imprecision of psychiatric diagnosis; nor is it easy to determine the beginning of a schizophrenic illness in a rather solitary and withdrawn adolescent in difficulty. In every one of these cases the treatment and the management are entirely different. Unless the general practitioner has qualified fairly recently, or has had some special experience in psychiatry, he is often likely to find himself at sea and in need of specialist advice. Often, too, his need is approved, encouraged, even accentuated by the patient himself, for the psychiatrist has that aura of the specialist so sought after today. He is now seldom, as he may once have been, either a figure to be feared or a figure of fun.

The expanding demand for out-patient treatment, the development of day hospitals and of in-patient units in general hospitals, and the care of the chronic patient in the community rather than in hospital have moved the centre of gravity of psychiatry and psychiatrists out of the mental hospital. In some fortunate areas a psychiatrist is employed jointly by the hospital service and by the local health authority and with his team looks after the mental health of a defined population. Elsewhere, particularly in big cities, the responsibility remains divided, areas overlap, the patients from a single borough may go to more than one hospital, a psychiatrist may treat patients from many boroughs and a few hospitals have no defined area from which they admit patients. In these conditions a smooth working relationship between the psychiatrist, the general practitioner and community workers is almost impossible to achieve. The people concerned cannot get to know each other well. The French, who have the same problem, estimate[1] that one psychiatrist with his team of three or more doctors should be able to look after the needs of 67,000 people. To cater for the needs of England and Wales on this scale the health service would need to employ the full time of 700 general psychiatric consultants. At present there are 860, but this number includes those involved in other branches—teaching, child guidance, special units, forensic psychiatry and so forth.

A Cure for All Ills

If psychiatry's recent progress in the treatment of psychotic illness is its most solid achievement to date—and the only one to appeal to those who prefer a scientific proof to a general impression—this is by no means the limit of its usefulness. A rich variety of new forms of treatment has sprung up, some of which are certainly effective. Others raise the question of what is "treatment", and also doubts about the bounds of medicine and the role of the psychiatrist in modern society.

Only in the field of subnormality—formerly called mental defect—has progress been slow. The old established methods hold. Delineation of the limits of the patient's capacity, supervision and support, training and occupation within those limits are the aims, either within an institution of some sort, or in a hostel, or at home. Prevention is appearing over the horizon. The simple screening of infants to detect phenylketonuria and the establishment of those who suffer from this metabolic abnormality on a special diet diminish the risk that they will become subnormal. The subtle technique of transfusing infants while they are still *in utero* may decrease the risk that Rhesus blood-group incompatibility between mother and unborn child will lead to kernicterus, a variety of mental defect.

General practitioners, increasingly alive to the possibility that their patients who complain of psychiatric, and some even who complain only of physical, symptoms can be helped by drugs, are coming to recognise how common an illness endogenous depression in fact is, and how easily treated. The same also holds true for many general physicians in hospital. Even some apparently neurotic patients respond to drug therapy, so that those clinicians who are most cautious about the *post hoc, ergo propter hoc* danger and more than suspicious of the effects of suggestion and placebos are having to

[1] *Europe et Santé*, (1963). WHO. Geneva.

change their opinions about the causes of some apparently neurotic
symptoms.

But what of the remaining neuroses, depressive states reactive to
circumstances and personality and behaviour disorders? These forms
of syndrome—it would be a mistake to use the word "disease" and
thereby imply known causes, a common course, a prognosis and
hopeful regime of treatment—are inextricably mixed. They consist
of mixtures of symptoms—depression, anxiety symptoms, obsessional
and compulsive symptoms, hysterical symptoms—occurring under
varying degrees of internal or external stress in personalities that are
usually abnormal in some way—anxious and obsessional, schizoid,
explosive, histrionic, phobic, inadequate or psychopathic. It is here
that psychiatrists differ most among themselves both about classification and about treatment; and it is here, too, that circular definition must offend[1] the logically minded critic and that psychiatry's
relations with morals continually cause trouble.

A huge array of treatment is available: psychotherapy in its
several forms; behaviour therapy; physical treatment including
drugs and surgery; manipulation of the environment.

Psychotherapy includes the various forms of analytical therapy,
which aim at bringing about a radical change in personality so that
the patient becomes more resistant to both internal and external
stresses. In the process he loses his symptoms and is enabled to deal
more effectively with further stress when he meets it. Psychotherapy
may be practised in groups and it may employ abreactive techniques
or hypnosis both as a means of exploration and for the removal of
symptoms. At the other extreme it may involve only sympathetic
listening, quite superficial advice and support and the cultivation
of a relationship between patient and therapist. Very often these,
coupled with some minor change at home, at work, or in social life,
are all that is required.

To some extent the psychiatrist has become heir to the general
practitioner as "guide, philosopher, and friend". Too many doctors
today have followed the scientific trend of orthodox medicine to
bother much about a patient who has neither physical signs of
illness nor abnormal laboratory findings; many feel uncomfortable
in this role and find it hard to believe that "just listening" can be
therapeutic; many are simply too busy, for listening requires time
and patience. The neurotic patient, too, has followed a trend. He

[1] In that, for example, "inadequate personality" as a nosological entity is defined as one
who is unable to deal adequately with the ordinary stresses of life. The "symptoms" of
this clinical entity are, in general, inability to deal adequately with ordinary stress.

reveres the expert even though in his case not much expertise is required. Theoretically, the patient's own doctor with his background knowledge of the patient, his family, and his situation should be better placed to fill this role. But many patients will only confess their problems to an outsider. This is understandable. "You seem more interested", "my doctor never has time", "I could never discuss this with my doctor", and "you never know who you will see" are remarks that tell of a malaise in general practice or at least of a changing pattern of medical care.

To some extent, too, the psychiatrist is nowadays heir to the parish priest. Statistics are hard to obtain that deal with church attendance in the last few decades. At least in towns and cities it seems to have declined, particularly for the young. To many, certainly, anything that smacks of religion is anathema and in difficulties people turn increasingly to medicine and to psychiatry. Priests confine their pastoral work to their flock of regular church attenders. The rest, who are not by any means necessarily irreligious, obtain social help through professional channels, of which psychiatry is one. As a result of the failure of what can be called a crash programme of pastoral work in Woolwich the vicar, then the Reverend Nicholas Stacey, concluded that priests should have a professional training in social work. Even active members of religious communities prefer sometimes to visit psychiatrists in their difficulties. The detachment and moral neutrality of the clinic make the discussion of impulses, wishes and conduct, about which they themselves have doubts or feelings of guilt, much simpler.

But is this medicine? Is it desirable that in this country psychiatric clinics, and in the United States psychoanalysts' offices, should be crowded with people whose need is for a confessor, a father-figure or a prop? Whether it is good or bad this is happening and it marks a change in the pattern of society.

Behaviour therapy is "the systematic application of principles derived from behaviour or learning theory, and the experimental work in these areas, to the rational modification of abnormal or undesirable behaviour".[1] It is rooted in the experimental techniques of Pavlov and his successors in Russia based on studies of conditioned reflexes, on the behaviourism of Watson, and on the learning theories of Hull and the animal ethologists. According to its exponents neurotic symptoms are caused by faulty unadaptive learning and

[1] Franks, C. M. *Conditioning Techniques in Clinical Practice and Research*. (Tavistock Publications. London, 1965).

conditioning, and psychopathic behaviour by deficient conditioning. Treatment of neurotic symptoms consists in the extinction of maladaptive learning, that is, unlearning or deconditioning, and treatment of psychopathic behaviour in the building up of desirable conditioned responses.[1] Much experimental work has been carried out on the various techniques of conditioning and deconditioning, and on many relevant constitutional factors such as individual variations in conditionability. Other subjects studied include the influence of drugs and of other environmental variables on the ease of conditioning and of extinction of conditioned responses.

Behaviour therapy is rooted in the science of experimental psychology, and a great deal of stress is laid by its exponents on proper scientific assessment of its results. It is a postwar development for the most part, and it is naturally too early yet for it to be evaluated as a valid and universally applicable successor to current methods of treating neurosis, most of which are in one way or another based on psychodynamic concepts.

Till now behaviour therapy's main successes have been with what can be called isolated neurotic symptoms—single phobias, stammering, fetishism, tics, writer's cramp, alcoholic addiction, bed-wetting —rather than with the commoner polysymptomatic neurotic conditions, and the reported results are impressive. But, so far, the literature of the subject has a scrappy look, a hotch-potch of reports of the treatment of a few cases of this and a handful of that. Unnecessary hostility, too, is often expressed by the authors to older systems of treatment, notably to analytical methods, and this invites retorts from those attacked. These counter-claim that as the behaviour therapist often spends a long time with his patients ferreting out details of their past history as well as in carrying out treatment a close emotional relationship must develop. This relationship, coupled with strong suggestion, accounts, they say, for the improvement or, more plausibly, it contributes an unknown amount to it. But it is not necessary that each side should disparage the efforts of the other. Brady and Lind[2] have, in fact, recorded a case of hysterical blindness treated successfully by "operant"[3] behaviour therapy. In the course of treatment phenomena occurred that strongly support the theory that the patient's symptom was a manifestation of repression and a

[1] Eysenck, H. J. ed. *Behaviour Therapy and the Neuroses*. (Pergamon Press. Oxford, 1960).
[2] Franks, C. M., op. cit.
[3] Operant, free-operant or instrumental conditioning refers to techniques in which the subject has to work, press buttons, pull levers to modify the situation, obtain rewards or avoid unpleasant consequences. It is contrasted with classical or Pavlovian conditioning in which he is a passive participant.

defence against anxiety. At several stages resistance was encountered to giving up the symptom and much anxiety reappeared.

Behaviour therapists have often been accused of being naïve and superficial and of removing symptoms only to leave the underlying illness untreated. They reply that the supposed danger—that in removing a symptom another worse one will appear instead—is unreal in their experience.

A worse accusation is of their association with "brainwashing". It is true that in the course of aversion treatment with emetic drugs for alcoholism or fetishism the patient becomes physically exhausted. In that state the patient is no doubt highly susceptible to the therapist's suggestions, just as the victim of brainwashing, exhausted by fear and lack of sleep, is suggestible to his captor's. But this is not the aim of the treatment and it does not happen during aversion deconditioning that employs electrical stimuli. The resemblance of behaviour therapy to brainwashing is superficial, and those who practise it can hardly be impugned on this account. Whether emetic drugs with all their dangers and unpleasantness should be employed by doctors is a different question.

This therapy is still in its infancy. We can confidently look forward to its developing more sophisticated techniques and perhaps to some success in finding ways to accelerate conditioning in those who are slow to develop social responses. Only then will psychology and psychiatry begin to be able to help in grappling with the bulk of delinquent behaviour.

The Limits

With the mention of delinquent behaviour and crime we again reach the limits of our subject. How much of it belongs to medicine—that is to psychiatry? This century has seen a steady increase in the amount of disordered behaviour which our society has been willing to regard as in the province of illness and treatment, and to detach from the realm of crime and punishment. The boundary fence has been steadily moved, pushed back, here a little there a little, with each new technique of investigation or treatment, and with the concept of diminished responsibility a new fence defining a no-man's-land has been set up.

Delinquent behaviour due to psychosis belongs, all agree, wholly to medicine. No one would think it right to imprison a confused and senile man who assaulted someone, or a woman who murdered her newborn baby when severely disturbed emotionally. Epilepsy arising from abnormality and injury to the temporal lobes of the brain, when it can be firmly diagnosed, is regarded as the medical cause of a few violent crimes. Severe depressives seldom commit crimes now that attempted suicide is no longer an offence, and the few schizophrenic patients who commit offences usually end up in hospital rather than in prison.

So far, so good. In children and young adolescents unhappiness and stress as often as not manifest themselves in disordered behaviour. The offences of children, when not dealt with purely medically by reference to the child psychiatrist and his team, are nearly always regarded as symptomatic of emotional disturbance in the child or his family or its substitute. They attract "treatment", in which the welfare of the child rather than the protection of society is the predominant aim.

Neurotic patients very seldom commit crimes unless there is in addition a character disorder. Society's methods of handling this last category of offender are at present irrational, inconsistent, sometimes unjust and cruel, often inadequate, and occasionally harmful or doomed to failure. Problems that are essentially similar may be dealt with quite capriciously either by the law—police, prison and probation officers—or by a psychiatrist, or by an uneasy combination of both. A man who steals feminine clothing from his neighbour's washing-line will probably be referred to a psychiatrist; one who goes out in the street in his wife's clothing may well go to prison. Someone who exposes himself to adolescent girls is often treated lightly, but two homosexuals found having sexual relations inconspicuously in a park may go to prison.

Insofar as there is rhyme or reason in all this, medicine tends to be allotted the following: those whose crimes are unexpected and unintelligible; the bizarre offenders who commit bizarre crimes; those who are young, meek and first offenders; many sexual offenders if the crime is not overtly aggressive; those who have been dealt with medically before.

Chaos and confusion reign in this twilight land between the sunlight of the "normal" offender and the clear moonlight of crime committed by someone who is obviously psychotic. All attempts by criminologists, doctors and social scientists to organise and systematise, to define and draw lines, have failed. No one has surpassed Lady Wootton in describing the present confusion.[1] After justly criticising the many current medical definitions of the psychopathic

[1] Wootton, B. *Social Science and Social Pathology.* (George Allen and Unwin. London, 1959).

personality which categorise him as sick—but which are also circular in that it is the antisocial behaviour that defines him as sick and yet the illness "explains" the antisocial behaviour—she sees no hope of holding a line of defence. "Revolutionary though the prospect of abandoning the concept of responsibility may be, it is clear that we are travelling steadily towards it" and "all intermediate positions . . . have shown themselves to be logically quite insecure." In effect, crime is on the way to becoming a disease.

Three inconsistent arguments, then, underlie present practice. Offenders who obviously suffer from some mental illness are dealt with in the province of medicine. The illness is seen as sufficient cause for the offence. If doctors can cure them well and good; if not, society expects them to keep the patient out of the general community. Offenders who are young are dealt with in keeping with their individual psychopathology and their individual needs in the hope that treatment, training or simple maturation will prevent a recurrence of their offences. In general society is tolerant of relapse. Offenders who are neither young nor psychotic are increasingly treated pragmatically. If there seems to be some hope that psychiatry can "cure" his condition the offender is regarded as a "patient" and handed over to the doctor for treatment; if not, the label "criminal" is attached and he remains within the arms of the law and its institutions. In contrast, however, to the policy of psychiatrists the criminal is released at the end of his sentence whether or not detention has had any beneficial effect. Indeed hardly anyone asks whether it has or has not.

Few moral philosophers, however, would go as far as Lady Wootton in abandoning the concepts of criminal responsibility, *mens rea*, and punishment. Professor Hart, for example, does not agree that the idea of responsibility is logically indefensible even if backward-looking ideas of relating the punishment to the crime are given up. ". . . I wish to reconsider the assumption . . . that only within the framework of a theory which sees punishment in a retributive and denunciatory light does the doctrine of responsibility make sense. There is, I believe, at this point something to defend, a moral position which ought not to be evacuated as if the decay of retributive ideas had made it untenable. There are values quite distinct from those of retributive punishment which the system of responsibility does maintain, and which remain of great importance even if our aims in punishing are the forward-looking aims of social protection."[1]

[1] Hart, H. L. A. *Punishment and the Elimination of Responsibility.* Hobhouse Memorial Lecture. (The Athlone Press of the University of London, London, 1962)

He appeals to common-sense: "If one person hits another the person struck does not think of the other as *just* a cause of pain to him; for it is of crucial importance to him whether the blow was deliberate or involuntary . . . If as our legal moralists maintain it is important for the law to reflect common judgements of morality, it is surely even more important that it should in general reflect in its judgements on conduct distinctions which not only underly [sic] morality but pervade the whole of our social life."

In another lecture published three years later[1] Professor Hart pleads for a moderate form of the new doctrine. In this thesis *mens rea* would continue to be a necessary condition of liability (with the usual qualifications about intention and age) to be decided before conviction, but the present qualification concerning mental abnormality would no longer obtain. It is plain that the divorce law in England has already moved in this direction. Since the decision in the House of Lords in *Gollins* v. *Gollins* in 1963 mental disorder has been no defence in divorce proceedings for cruelty.

Mental abnormality, according to Professor Hart, should be assessed only after conviction so that appropriate "treatment"can be prescribed. On this point he and Lady Wootton are in agreement.

Two other points are worth making. First, if punishment and treatment are to be equated, and if no treatment is likely to be successful for one who has committed a fairly trivial offence, it might seem outrageous to keep him in custody for the rest of his life. Some psychiatrists do just this in a few cases of, say, chronic schizophrenia. Secondly, community care, considered by doctors to be so important in the management of the incompletely recovered psychotic, is minimal for ex-prisoners, and after-care and follow-up hardly exist for most of them.

The present confusion is symptomatic of a deeper rift. The dominant psychologies of the present time, psychoanalysis and behaviourism, are determinist. They seek causality in the phenomena of human behaviour just as scientists have been seeking it so successfully in the world of inanimate things. Our society and we ourselves as individuals do not accept a thoroughgoing determinism as the sole explanation of human behaviour. To ourselves we appear to have free will and in its attitude to its members society concurs. Indeed the Existentialists and the Roman Catholics are almost alone among modern psychiatrists in believing that the essence of human nature is the power of choosing freely. Motives, aims, intentions,

[1] Hart, H. L. A. *Changing Conceptions of Responsibility.* Lionel Cohen Lectures. Magnes Press. (The Hebrew University. Jerusalem, 1965).

purposes express a reality of our own, and presumably therefore of other human, experience. Nevertheless the study of psychotic behaviour, experiments with drugs and sensory deprivation, research into the electrophysiology of the brain, and analysis of human behaviour in groups are some of the forces in the tide of scientific knowledge that is eroding the concept of free will. Will it in the course of time, like a sandcastle, disappear altogether?

In the course of this century the psychiatrist's role has expanded, like his subject, tremendously. Previously only a guardian of the insane he has now become in turn a diagnostician and a scientist, an educator of parents, a confessor, a clinician in general hospitals, a supporter for the unhappy, a mediator between husband and wife, a job-selector, a father-figure, a social scientist and social worker, an agent of preventive medicine, and an arbiter between punishment and treatment. It is not surprising that he has sometimes, too, become a scapegoat for the ills of society.

CHAPTER EIGHT

General Theories of Disease

Division and Unity in Medicine

The previous chapters from science to psychiatry have shown how the span of medicine has progressively widened in this century. At one extreme in intensive care units and in transplant surgery the richly growing resources of scientific medicine are focused, as by a lens, on the individual patient and his disease; next, in preventive medicine the effort is diffused from an individual to a population, and more widely still to solving medical problems on a world scale; then in geriatric medicine the scope has expanded further, for here doctors must often deal with multiple disease and disabilities in an individual whose total illness cannot be effectively treated unless its social and economic framework is taken into account; lastly, at the other extreme is psychiatry where at the limits medicine merges with pedagogy, criminology, religion and moral philosophy, and where disease, often enough, has become a meaningless question-begging word.

It is almost miraculous that with super-specialists digging deeper in ever-narrowing seams and other specialists ranging ever more widely and crossing boundaries into other disciplines medicine has not cracked wide open. To some extent it has in every advanced country (in Britain the built-in tripartitism of its health service has been a special flaw); to some extent language, concepts and theories have become so esoteric as to bar communication.

Fortunately, however, powerful unifying forces are at work and a dialogue is still possible. There are trends in medical education, for example, tending to delay specialisation. There are the teams derived from several disciplines engaged in therapy and research. Both the continuing strength of general medical journals and the extension of medical journalism to the lay press help to preserve unity, for doctors now are near-laymen in all medical subjects but their own.

But the strongest tendency favouring unity arises from medicine's remaining, in the hackneyed phrase, art as well as science. In treating their patients doctors have to act before the causes of disease are fully known. They have a need for open hypotheses, for theories that can be adapted as scientific knowledge grows.

This chapter is devoted to aetiological theory and surveys three of this century's most pervasive general hypotheses of disease: psychosomatic disorder, stress disease and auto-immunity. These theories are now undoubtedly in the stage of overinclusiveness before being cut down to size. They overlap and they range from the extreme of psychological to the extreme of physical interpretation.

Just as doctors in their practice have clutched at remedies that, aided by the placebo-effect and the doctors' own enthusiasm, have seemed for a time to work wonders till disillusion has set in, so too they have grasped at general theories of disease and applied them to any disease of unknown cause. The art of medicine is littered therefore with discarded remedies and with theories which, if not abandoned, have in the course of time contracted to embrace only what continues to be useful. For medicine is science as well as art, and Bernard Shaw little thought that he was paying medicine a compliment when he wrote:

"Medical theories are so much a matter of fashion, and the most fertile of them are modified so rapidly by medical practice and biological research ... that the play [*The Doctor's Dilemma*] ... is already slightly out-moded."

Examples of overinclusive theories or, one should perhaps say, of the overenthusiastic use of theories in this century, of theories that have now been cut down to size, are the germ theory, allergy and focal sepsis. These are no longer fertile.

Organised medicine, its plasticity preserved by advances in the basic sciences, behaves better, in this respect, than the branches of what has been called "fringe medicine". These cults, based on single theories—osteopathy, acupuncture, radiesthesia, naturopathy, Christian Science, homeopathy and the rest—are closed systems, rooted in unshakable faith and impervious to arguments based on scientific evidence. Their chief champion in Britain and, since Shaw, orthodox medicine's most voluble and persuasive critic, Mr Inglis,[1] claims the opposite to be true: "the medical profession today resembles one of those primeval monsters who were efficiently armoured against dinosaurs and other predators but helpless when confronted with a change of climate." The uncommitted person can safely be left to

[1] Inglis, Brian. *Fringe Medicine*. (Faber and Faber. London, 1964).

judge which is the more unadaptable. Mr Inglis asserts, moreover, that there is a current revival of fringe medicine. He does not produce a shred of evidence that this is so. It seems unlikely.

The Psychosomatic Hypothesis

In its broadest form this theory merely restates what is axiomatic to everyone who is not a Cartesian dualist: that in all illness there must be both psychic and somatic elements and that any division of medicine into "physical" and "mental" categories is logically indefensible. It is salutary for everyone to recall from time to time that all classification of this kind necessarily involves error and over-simplifies the phenomena of illness. In practice it can be rewarding in treating a neurotic illness, an anxiety state, say, to recall that the patient may not be improving with psychological methods of treatment because he is grossly underweight or anaemic. Equally, someone with a predominantly physical illness, such as pulmonary tuberculosis, may not respond properly to physical methods of treatment because she has anxieties about the future or about the welfare of her children. There are limits, of course, to the relevance of this kind of approach and there are practical limits too. A young man of twenty fractures a leg in a motor-cycle accident. His leg heals well and he returns to work. Would it be good preventive medicine to ask why he crashed? Was he going too fast and vying with a friend? Why did he have this powerful machine at all? A series of questions in endless recession taking enquiry back to the womb and before. To answer them adequately would require a full psychiatric and social history, interviews with the parents, perhaps a school report and so forth.

All illness has many causes and enquiry into the less obvious ones can sometimes be rewarding; it can show reasons why one person suffers from a certain disease and another fails to respond quickly to treatment. In the enlarging fields of accidents, both accident-proneness and the compensation situation are elements that most people today would consider relevant. Accidents in the home, venereal disease, the personality characteristics of people involved in road traffic accidents and of heavy smokers are examples of other parts of the field of illness where psychosomatic research could be valuable.

But the word is more often used in a restricted sense to apply to a group of illnesses and groups of symptoms that lie between the two extremes of "pure" psychiatric and physical disease. They have some characteristics in common: they are chronic and, now that infectious illness is to a great extent under control, becoming more important in medicine; until lately they have usually been considered medical rather than psychiatric; their causes have long been suspected of being complex but remain largely unknown. The list of disorders is quite long, and most doctors who accept the concept at all would include most or all of the following: asthma, especially in adult life; duodenal and perhaps gastric ulceration; rheumatoid arthritis; hypertension and perhaps coronary artery disease; hyperthyroidism; certain skin diseases in addition to neurodermatitis; possibly ulcerative colitis; certainly migraine and dysmenorrhoea.

People who support the psychosomatic hypothesis say that there are important (though not exclusive) psychic causes for these illnesses which have long been ignored. These causes derive from morbid emotion, which has been shown by Pavlov, Cannon and others to be capable of influencing every organ of the body and every bodily function. A persistent disturbance of some bodily function may result in structural damage. Supporters of the theory have to probe deeply so that they can attempt to answer certain crucial questions about the illness. Why, for instance, did it happen to this particular patient? Why did this morbid emotion manifest itself in this organ or system and not in that? Why did the illness happen when it did? They make use of subsidiary concepts, many derived from dynamic psychological theory but many that are not, such as conditioning. They try to produce a coherent explanation which interprets the patient's life history, emotional problems, relationships, needs and experiences in terms of established physiology and psychology to answer the why, when and where questions about his symptoms.

A vast literature of the subject has accumulated in the last forty years or so. In one of her books[1] Dr Flanders Dunbar gives a list of over 5,000 references. Much of this work is open to criticism, and the whole theory is hardly one that appeals to scientists, for rigorous enquiry is barely possible in this field. In the first place much of the work is anecdotal, a description of a few cases of a particular disease with the author's plausible interpretation and an account of his efforts at treatment, more or less successful, along psychotherapeutic lines. Secondly, there are few studies that incorporate a control group. Thirdly, many of the enthusiasts are defensive and polemical, quite often unprepared to admit that even if the main cause of a disease is commonly emotional there may be other causes at work in many

[1] Dunbar, Flanders. *Emotion and Bodily Changes.* (Columbia University Press. New York, 1954).

patients and that in some patients emotion may not be important at all. Fourthly, there is an unwillingness to admit that even if an account is plausible it is not necessarily true. Fifthly, the results of treatment based on the hypothesis have not, it must be admitted, been very impressive; but they have been quite often good enough to make it likely that in *some* patients with *some* of these diseases the doctor was on the right track. The results in asthma, certain skin troubles and migraine are on the whole better than in the others; however, the enthusiast for psychosomatic medicine can defend himself by saying that if functional disorder has proceeded to structural change, treatment is much more difficult. Lastly, many generalisations have gone too far. Some authors have forced all their clinical material into a mould of their own making. The result has come out looking so monotonous in form that one suspects that it tells one more about the mould than about the material that went into it. For example Dr Flanders Dunbar in her immense study[1] of more than 1,200 admissions to hospital with fractures, diabetes and cardiovascular diseases produces personality profiles for people who suffer from these and other conditions. Of diabetics she says: "these patients appear distant and reserved, wavering between tentative friendly gestures and suspicious withdrawal . . . they are generally inhibited and their reaction under emotional stress has the all or none quality of the infant." This, presumably, is a description which is meant to fit the personalities of the 600,000 or so Americans who at any one time are disabled by this disease. She goes farther than this in approving Dr Walter Alvarez's generalisation about stomach-ulcers occurring in the "go-getter" type. She labels patients who suffer from coronary artery disease "top-dogs", hypertensives "would be top-dogs", people with rheumatic fever and rheumatic heart disease "teacher's pets and martyrs", and diabetics "muddlers". These generalisations are as useless, unscientific and dangerous as the stereotypes of nations and classes that bedevil so much social and political thinking.

Absurd overgeneralisation of this kind has tended to bring into disrepute the methods and discoveries, indeed the whole approach, of psychosomatic medicine. This is a pity because they have been and continue to be fruitful in the understanding of many patients and their illnesses. In fact, medicine cannot afford to discard the psychosomatic theory. It is too valuable and contains a lot of truth but not the whole truth. Perhaps it will soon permeate the approach of ordinary doctors to their patients with these common diseases.

[1] Dunbar, Flanders. *Psychosomatic Diagnosis.* (Paul B. Hoeber. New York, 1943).

If it does it will be thanks to the energy and persuasiveness of those enthusiasts who in the last thirty years have fought for a hearing.

If psychosomatic theory is the most psychological of the three chosen theories, the next, the stress hypothesis, is the most all-embracing.

The Stress Hypothesis

It is most unfortunate that the words "stress", "stress reaction" and "stress disease" should mean so many different things to different people. To physiologists stress means the state of an animal (including human beings) produced by a variety of agents, physical, toxic, bacterial, emotional; to some doctors the word is equivalent to emotional stress or intrapsychic conflict, and the stress disorders are equivalent to psychosomatic diseases; to others it means particular changes in the environment; some use the words precisely and define them rigidly; others say that they know what the words mean but that, like pain, they are indefinable. The confusion is highly unsatisfactory and, as has so often happened before in biology, new words are needed rather than old words enlarged.

One who has defined the words most carefully of all to the extent of almost making them his own is Dr Hans Selye. In 1946 after many years of animal research he first published his general theory of stress,[1] and in many publications from his Institute at McGill University, Montreal, he has extended and elaborated it. A well-known British doctor, Sir Heneage Ogilvie, has described his work as "perhaps the greatest contribution to scientific medicine in this century"—a formidable claim—and perhaps in consequence the theory is very difficult to describe succinctly yet accurately.

As an outcome of his animal experiments Dr Selye described his fundamental concept, the general adaptation syndrome (GAS), a specific syndrome activated nonspecifically by a host of stressful agents additional to any local damage that they might do. The agents include heat, cold, toxins, exertion, injury, invasion by bacteria, frustration and rage, and the injection of foreign protein. The GAS as so described comprises three phases: the alarm reaction, the stage of resistance, and the stage of exhaustion. The alarm reaction, "a generalised call to arms of the defensive forces of the body", is produced only by agents that have a general effect on large portions of the body. It derives more from the extent of the attack than from its local intensity. Unless the agent is so damaging

[1] Selye, H. (1946), *J.Clin. Endocrinol.*, **6**, 117.

L

that it causes death in a few hours or a day or two the alarm reaction is succeeded by the stage of resistance, of which the bodily manifestations are quite different, often indeed the opposite. The three primary bodily changes of the alarm reaction are enlargement of the adrenals; shrinkage of the lymphatic structures, thymus, spleen and lymph nodes; and the appearance of bleeding gastro-duodenal ulceration. In addition eosinophil cells tend to disappear from the blood, sodium is retained, potassium is lost, and there is loss of weight. In the succeeding stage of resistance most of these changes are reversed and this stage of adaptation persists until the stressor is removed, infection overcome, or repair is in progress.

If exposure to serious harm persists, however, the stage of exhaustion may supervene; then, many of the chemical, metabolic and cellular changes are reversed once more when the organism is *in extremis* before death.

On the basis, again, of his animal experiments, Selye became convinced that these phases of his syndrome were mediated by alterations in the amounts and balance of hormones[1] put out by the pituitary and consequently by the cortex (or rind) of the adrenal glands. These hormones produce much longer-lasting effects than adrenaline, the hormone of the adrenal medulla (or core), which, as was established long ago, is poured out in immediately alarming situations and reinforces the preparations for fight-or-flight made by the autonomic[2] nervous system. The hormones concerned in the pituitary–adrenal axis that are concerned in the adaptation syndrome are many, but broadly they can be assigned, he says, to two opposing groups:

a. the pituitary adrenocorticotrophic hormone (ACTH), which induces the cortex of the suprarenal to make increased amounts of glucocorticoids[3] (such as cortisol). These hormones diminish inflam-

---

[1] Hormones, the exceedingly potent chemicals secreted directly into the blood stream by the endocrine glands—the pituitary, thyroid, adrenals, pancreas, parathyroids, ovaries and testes. They act on distant parts of the body. Many of the pituitary hormones act upon the other endocrine glands and as part of a homeostatic (negative feed-back) mechanism the hormones of these other glands themselves act upon the pituitary. Thus, an increase in circulating cortisol from the cortex of the adrenal inhibits the secretion of the pituitary adrenocorticotrophic hormone (ACTH), which stimulates the adrenal cortex to pour out cortisol. This is the reason why cortisone given by mouth, say, in a case of rheumatoid arthritis causes reduced activity of the patient's own adrenals.

[2] Autonomic: sympathetic and parasympathetic nervous system. This system is especially concerned with the control of involuntary muscles, the calibre of blood vessels, the motility and emptying of hollow viscera such as the stomach and the bladder, and sweating. It is closely concerned with the bodily changes that accompany emotion.

[3] Glucocorticoids, a group of adrenal cortical hormones with prominent effects on glucose metabolism; contrasted with minerala-corticoids which specially influence salt metabolism.

nation, raise blood-sugar, lessen allergic reactions, raise blood
pressure and favour bleeding from the gastro-intestinal tract.
2. the pituitary somatotrophic hormone (STH, growth hormone),
which acts on tissues itself directly but which also in all probability
encourages the secretion of mineralocorticoids (such as aldosterone
and deoxycorticosterone) from the suprarenal cortex. These hormones are pro-inflammatory, encourage the excretion of potassium
and the retention of sodium.

Selye, himself, recognises that this simple grouping oversimplifies
the facts[1] and that in many respects these two groups of hormones
are not antagonistic, for example in favouring sodium retention and
potassium excretion. Some critics, however, while acknowledging an
ACTH–adrenal cortical axis, say that the evidence for a growth
hormone–adrenal cortical axis is scanty. The mode of action of
growth hormone is ill-understood, but it has not been shown to have
any direct effect on the secretion of either aldosterone or deoxycorticosterone which, in any case, are not usually described as pro-
inflammatory.

Diseases of adaptation, Selye believes, are caused, or partly caused,
by imperfections in the working of this system. Many diseases seem
to be due less to the direct results of the environment, injury, infection
and the like, than to the body's inability to adapt itself properly to
these threats. Diseases which there is reason to think are at least partly
caused by faults in adaptation include the rheumatic diseases, peptic
ulceration, allergic disorders, hypertension and arterial degeneration,
and some varieties of diabetes and hyperthyroidism.

The main conclusions of Selye's research and thought have been
generally accepted, though there is much criticism of detail. Not
many people have followed him beyond his general theory of adaptation, and the diseases of adaptation, into the realms where he dis-
cusses "adaptation energy", ageing, "reactions", and his philosophy.
The validity of his views is most obvious in conditions such as surgical
shock, severe injuries, and extensive burns, where a great deal of
damage has been inflicted in a short time. Professor Butterfield,[2][3]
for example, studied twenty severely burned patients and found low
sodium excretion, a fall in eosinophil white blood cells, increased
excretion of adrenal cortical hormones, glucose in the urine and other
changes that would be expected if Selye's theories are valid. One

---

[1] Selye, H. *The Stress of Life.* (Longmans, Green. London, 1957).
[2] Evans, E. I., and Butterfield, W. J. H. (1951), *Ann. Surg.*, **134,** 588.
[3] Butterfield, W. J. H. in *The Nature of Stress Disorder.* (Hutchinson Medical Publications. London, 1959).

elderly woman even became persistently diabetic. The changes were proportional to the extent of the burn. It is less firmly established that milder insults acting over a longer time would give rise to similar chemical and metabolic abnormalities in human beings.

This very extensive research on animals, and the theories arising from it, even if one has to bear in mind that there are notable differences in response between species, at least gives a hint of the mechanism by which emotion, shocking experiences, long-continued tension, and inhibited aggressive urges might produce the so-called stress diseases. Those doctors who have long been convinced from their own observations that attacks of asthma, exacerbations of peptic ulceration, breakdown of tuberculosis, and eruptions of skin disorders are provoked by excess of emotional tension have at least most of the possible pathways mapped out. Here, at last, the two extreme definitions of "stress diseases" come within sight of each other. At one pole there is the group of illnesses of which a major cause is emotional disturbance. They begin at a time of crisis, they fluctuate in keeping with the degree of emotional disturbance, and they clear up when either the situation changes for the better or the patient learns to adapt to it without undue tension.[1] At the other, there are the maladies in which imperfections of the general adaptation syndrome play a role. Many kinds of agent can call up these defences: emotional disturbance may be one.

The third general theory is intensely physical, although it has been used in partial explanation of the origin of some of the psychoses.

The Hypothesis of Auto-immune Disease

This new and pervasive concept describes a group of illnesses in which it seems probable that the main cause, or at least a contributory cause, is a fault in the mechanism that ordinarily ensures that the immunity defences of the body only attack "foreign" substances. These defences have developed to repel invasion by bacteria and to neutralise bacterial toxins. As the toxins and the coats of bacteria are both composed of protein the defence mechanisms are alerted by any invasion of the body by protein from whatever source, even if the protein is that of a harmless pollen in the mucous membrane of the nose or that of a horse inevitably accompanying an injection of tetanus antitoxin prepared from that animal. Anything that will evoke an antibody-response is termed an antigen and most antigens

[1] O'Neill, D. in *The Nature of Stress Disorder.*

are protein in nature. When one speaks of invasion of the body it is the tissues of the body that are concerned and not the lumen of the gastro-intestinal tract, which for this purpose has to be regarded as a hollow tube that the body surrounds but which is not part of the body. Antibody is not developed to fillet steak in the stomach, but it would be were the steak to be injected.

In auto-immune disease there seems to be a failure on the part of the immunity defences of the body to distinguish self from not-self. Damage is caused by the cells of the antibody-producing system and by antibodies attacking normal components of the body, mistaking them for "foreign".

It has been known for a very long time that the processes determining immunity to foreign material can go wrong occasionally and by their excess give rise to such troublesome conditions as asthma, hay-fever, eczema and serum sickness. What is new is the hypothesis that there can be equally damaging consequences from faults in the original labelling system. If this happens, "self" cells may years later be treated as "foreign" and destroyed. A further source of auto-immune disease is a mutation in a cell that forms antibodies, with the effect that this cell's progeny, which have multiplied in the body, react against normal body cells.

The capacity to make antibodies in response to antigens seems to appear quite late in foetal life. There continues to be controversy about the mechanism. According to one set of theories the maturing animal contains a very large range of antibody-producing cells, each of which is capable of giving rise to only one kind of antibody. When a specific antigen enters the body, say, some measles virus when the child is five, it will soon chance to encounter the appropriate cell, which is selectively stimulated to produce anti-measles antibody, whereas all the thousands of other defensive cells will ignore the presence of this virus. This cell's descendants, termed a "clone", will continue to produce this antibody or have the potentiality to do so. This view of what happens is incorporated in the clonal selection hypothesis of Burnet. Late in foetal life, Burnet suggests, at the time when the capacity to form antibodies first emerges, all those clones of cells that are capable of reacting with "self" antigens, one's own proteins, are destroyed. Only those which are incapable of self-reaction survive. For this purpose "self" includes the antigens of an identical twin, for these must be identical as their genetic constitution is the same. It includes, too, the antigens of a fraternal twin that shared the same placenta, for mixing of blood must have occurred at this stage of foetal life. It includes also, as Sir Peter Medawar's[1] experiments have shown, the antigens of any animal of the same species whose living cells were injected into the foetus before birth.

The other group of theories suggests that every cell of the antibody-producing system is capable of producing an antibody appropriate to any antigen that it encounters. The response of such a cell is determined not by its genetic qualities but by the "instruction" which the antigen provides. This group of "instructive" theories assumes that tolerance to "self" antigens is maintained by the persistence of these antigens in antibody-forming cells or in cells in close relationship to them.

Both "selective" and "instructive" theories have their advantages and their difficulties and neither is yet universally accepted.

The phenomena of auto-immune disease stem from the emergence of cells which are able to react with "self" components and produce antibody against them. These groups of cells have been called by Burnet[2] "forbidden clones". They may arise in at least two ways. First, a mutation may occur which endows that cell and its descendants with the capacity to produce antibodies. Secondly, certain antigens do not ordinarily come into contact with antibody-producing cells at the critical time in foetal life when self-reacting cells are destroyed. These include thyroglobulin, which is locked away in storage in the thyroid gland, lens tissue, which has negligible blood supply, and spermatozoa, which are stored in the epididymis and seminal vesicles and to which blood cells have little or no access. These antigens are termed "inaccessible". Those clones which can react with their protein antigens do not get destroyed but persist, and if they gain access to these inaccessible antigens later in life can do damage. These are two of the ways in which it is thought that "forbidden clones" and auto-antibodies can arise.

The agents causing auto-immune disease, therefore, are two: immunologically competent cells which can travel to target organs and there produce damage; and circulating auto-antibody.

A number of criteria needs to be satisfied before a disease can confidently be regarded as auto-immune in aetiology; these are stated by Burnet[3] to comprise the following:

1. A high gammaglobulin level in the blood plasma. It is with this

---

[1] Medawar, P. B. *The Immunology of Transplantation*. Harvey Lectures. (Academic Press. New York, 1956).
[2] Burnet, F. M. (1959), *Brit. Med. J.*, **ii,** 645 and 720.
[3] Mackay, I. R. and Burnet, F. M. *Auto-immune Diseases*. (Charles C. Turner. Springfield, Illinois, 1963).

fraction of the blood plasma proteins that antibody activity is closely associated.

2. The presence of auto-antibody against a normal body constituent: antibodies which agglutinate blood cells—rheumatoid factor, and lupus erythematosus factor, for example.

3. Deposition of altered gammaglobulin in certain tissues such as the kidney.

4. Accumulations of lymphocytes in the tissues of target organs. These are the cells that are doing active damage by producing auto-antibody.

5. At least a partial response to corticosteroid drugs such as cortisone and its newer derivatives. A response to these drugs does not in itself suggest that a disease is auto-immune, for they are, of course, of great value in treating disorders of immunity, such as asthma and some eczemas, in which the antigen is foreign and not "self".

6. Evidence that some other auto-immune process is going on at the same time.

In addition, there is usually a suggestion that genetic factors are at work, and there is a curious and unexplained tendency for females to be affected more commonly than males by these illnesses.

At the present time this is an active growing point in medicine, and a vast literature is accumulating. Almost every week there are reports of research indicating, confirming, or denying that auto-immune factors have been found to be operating in some new field. The situation changes, therefore, from month to month. It appears to be quite certain that three diseases, all uncommon, are of auto-immune origin—Hashimoto's thyroiditis, systemic lupus erythematosus and a group of haemolytic anaemias. Most people would add pernicious anaemia to this group. There is strong evidence that auto-immune processes are playing a large part in causing a group of other illnesses, many of them much commoner: rheumatoid arthritis and the so-called collagen diseases; myasthenia gravis; some types of encephalitis; many cases both of myxoedema and hyperthyroidism; one type of male sterility; and some diseases of the lens, the iris, and the ciliary body of the eye. The evidence is as yet much less complete that auto-immune processes are of more than slight importance in such fairly common conditions as ulcerative colitis, multiple sclerosis, nephritis, and rheumatic fever. There is even some hope that this fertile theory and the extremely complex methods of investigation developed in connection with it will prove useful in eventually un-ravelling the causes of cancer and of ageing.

Aetiological Theory

A lesson that needs emphasising and that Bernard Shaw altogether missed is that these general theories are fertile precisely because they are open and adaptable; they unify because for a time at least too much is claimed; no doubt excessive claims are irritating, but in so being they generate further research.

In trying to treat illnesses of unknown cause doctors are happier with implausible hypotheses than with none at all. As each new general theory of disease is suggested it is, as it were, tried on for size. Does it fit cases of multiple sclerosis? Can it accommodate the facts of ulcerative colitis?

But of all the remaining problems of aetiology the cause or causes of rheumatoid arthritis are at once the most familiar and the most baffling.

At the turn of the century insofar as this condition was distinguished from other varieties of "rheumatism"—rheumatic fever, subacute rheumatism and osteoarthritis—its cause was either frankly admitted to be unknown or attributed to a "diathesis", which was a circular definition. It defined the cause of rheumatoid arthritis as a permanent constitutional liability of the body to get the disease.

By the 1930s the prevailing view, supported by much evidence, was that the disease was infective in origin and it was customary to hunt in every case for foci of infection in teeth, sinuses, tonsils and gall bladder or elsewhere and to eradicate them. Some time later, largely because actual organisms could so seldom be found in the affected joints, the focal sepsis theory was modified. It was suggested either that the disease was caused by toxins absorbed from a focus of infections or that the organisms produced a sensitisation of the joint and other tissues concerned and that the arthritis was in fact an allergic manifestation.

Meanwhile endocrine disorder, dietary deficiency and some mysterious metabolic anomaly such as underlies gout had been suggested and rejected. Needless to say, regimes of treatment based on all these theories, the eradication of septic foci, a warm climate, and special diets, all had their successes, but for the majority they failed to cure or even to relieve.

Twenty years or so ago the theory that rheumatoid arthritis was a psychosomatic disorder began to gain ground. Studies were made of the influence of emotional stress in causing the illness, or at least in provoking exacerbations, and of the type of personality which was vulnerable. As usual, a voluminous literature steadily accumulated, but the results of treatment by psychological methods were in general disappointing.

In 1948 Hench's discovery that cortisone dramatically relieved the severe joint symptoms of the disease for a time revolutionised treatment. The cause seemed to be on the point of discovery, but the drug's side-effects, its capacity to produce psychological dependence and its failure as a long-term therapy were a profound disappointment. Nevertheless the ability of adrenal cortical hormones to suppress symptoms at least indicated the kind of pathway along which emotional stress could operate in those cases where the disease could convincingly be shown to be psychosomatic.

The evidence that rheumatoid arthritis is an auto-immune disease also dates from 1948. In that year Rose[1] and other workers confirmed an experiment first reported by Waaler[2] and identified a "rheumatoid factor" in the serum of patients suffering from the disease. In the mysterious and highly technical language of immunology these sera "agglutinate sheep cells coated with a subagglutinating dose of rabbit anti-sheep cell antiserum".[3] This rheumatoid factor is present in about 90% of patients, but about 10% of cases run their full course without developing it. It is present in other auto-immune diseases, notably in some cases of systemic lupus erythematosus, and in nature it appears, surprisingly, to be an anti-antibody, that is, an antibody to the patient's own gammaglobulin. The evidence that rheumatoid arthritis is an auto-immune disease rests partly on the finding of this factor in a high proportion of cases but on other evidence too. The factor occurs more frequently in the relatives of rheumatoid patients than in controls; the disease occurs predominantly in females; there is a high level of gammaglobulin in the blood particularly when the disease is active; there is deposition of altered globulin in the rheumatoid nodules; the lining membrane of the affected joints contains dense masses of lymphoid cells, which make the rheumatoid factor as demonstrated by the technique of immuno-fluorescence. The illness responds at least partially to corticosteroid drugs; and it not uncommonly occurs in association with other undoubted auto-immune diseases. However, in spite of much weight

[1] Rose, H. W., Ragan, C., Pearce, E., and Lipman, M. O. (1948), *Proc. Soc. Exper. Biol. Med.*, **68**, 1.
[2] Waaler, E. (1940). *Acta Path. Microbiol. Scandinav.*, **17**, 172.
[3] Glynn, L. E. and Holborrow, E. J. *Autoimmunity and Disease.* (Blackwell Scientific Publications, Oxford, 1965).

of evidence there remain several technical difficulties to be disposed of before this disease can be accepted unequivocally as being of auto-immune origin.

At the moment these two general theories of disease, the psychosomatic (and "stress") and the auto-immune, are the most versatile hypotheses medicine possesses for exploring several of its unknown tracts. To some extent their fields of relevance overlap: in rheumatoid arthritis, for example, and in accounting for the significance of the effects of corticosteroids; less confidently in ulcerative colitis, hyperthyroidism, and the vast kidney-hypertension-arterial degeneration complex. It is unfortunate that the two theories seem to be so irreconcilable and that their adherents at best ignore each other. No doubt the excess of plausibility and lack of controlled studies of the one are as infuriating to some people as the ultra-scientific materialism of the second is to others.

Presumably we are standing too close to the problem so that the two aspects cannot be in the field of vision at the same time. To a policeman London's traffic problem must largely be a matter of parked cars and empty buses. He is not concerned with more distant causes. But to a planner the drift of an increasingly rich population to the south-east of England may be a more obvious and basic cause. In medicine the aetiology of most of the diseases that have single predominating causes—infections, deficiencies, genetic metabolic disorders—must by now have been worked out. Perhaps a few remain to be discovered and, certainly, the search must continue, just as it must go on for secondary causes for such conditions as tuberculosis, accidents, or lung cancer, of which the prime cause is known. But more and more the concept of multiple aetiology, of combining and contributory causation, seems to fit the facts best. As has been accepted for a long time in psychiatry, a "diagnosis" can no longer be usefully expressed in one, two or three words. It more often needs a sentence or two if it is to serve the primary purpose of diagnosis and prescribe a likely course, a probable outcome, and useful therapy. Perhaps the same stage has been reached in diabetes, in rheumatoid arthritis, arterial degeneration and chronic bronchitis. In these and many other illnesses it seems futile to hunt for a prime cause as the preponderant cause in all cases. It is more constructive to assess the individual's illness in terms of a number of "causes" that may be concurrent, consecutive or interlocking—genetic and constitutional, infective, dietary, social, traumatic, emotional, auto-immune and so forth. This concept is not new, but the startling success of the "single cause" outlook in this century, its triumphs in infections, deficiencies of diet, and biochemical disorders, and its mechanistic simplicity and clarity seemed to make anything more complicated unnecessary. Does insulin solve all the problems of diabetes? Is tuberculosis caused by the tubercle bacillus and cured by streptomycin and other drugs? Is rheumatic fever caused by the haemolytic streptococcus and its sequels by this organism's toxin? Is obesity caused by eating too much and cured by dieting? The answers to all these questions are yes in a sense, but only in a very limited sense. Medicine is seldom so simple and straightforward as they imply.

Scientists may burrow, each in his own corner, and from time to time come up with brilliant discoveries and occasionally with great unifying concepts, but discoveries and fresh concepts do not of necessity invalidate all that has gone before. In solving the great remaining puzzles—cancer, ageing, degenerations of arteries and in the central nervous system, and neurosis—medicine will have need for all that discovery can offer. Unless more is discarded from the present pool of knowledge than seems possible it is likely, too, to need to revive the concept of multifactorial aetiology.

CHAPTER NINE

Frontier Medicine

It is usual to think of the word disease as implying a naturally occurring disorder. So far, in this book, the discussion has been largely confined to natural diseases or to the prevention of them in healthy people even when, as in the chapter on psychiatry, the word disease has been stretched beyond its ordinary meaning. Even the iatrogenic diseases, though caused by doctors, at least arise from efforts to treat natural disease. The exception, some of the consequences of experimental medicine, has aroused criticism, as we have seen, on ethical grounds; these criticisms arise because doctors have taken unjustified risks with other people's health in the interests of science.

But increasingly in this century people take risks with their own health. Aided by twentieth century technology and by engines of various kinds they try to go farther, faster, higher and deeper than ever before, and in doing so usually attract praise and admiration unless they are too foolhardy. If, like Icarus, they fly too high doctors pick up the bits. The urge to explore must be as old as man himself; indeed, as a characteristic of animals in general, it must always have been one of the main instruments of natural selection. Perhaps it still is. Perhaps, in spite of the obvious virtue of meekness and conformity in our crowded Western societies the adventurous still get the best girls. In recent centuries other motives, economic and strategic, for example, have been grafted on to the basic drive that is so inadequately termed curiosity. In our century competitive sport, with its stakes recently raised by the century's most successful political movement—nationalism—has provided a great stimulus to exploration. But today, in this as in so many other fields, it is war and preparation for war, the fear of being outflanked on this frontier, that provide the chief motive.

Medicine has been involved in exploration ever since their journeys brought men up against physiological barriers—desert heat, polar cold, and the thin air of high altitudes. Increasingly in this century since men invaded the depths of the sea, the air, and now space, it has been the physiological frontiers, the capacity of men to survive and work in these abnormal environments, that have set the limit to exploration.

The information that a manned expedition can gather in comparison with any other kind, either purely mechanical or one employing animals, is so superior in amount and quality that an immense effort in physiological research has been made. The limits of human tolerance to various physical stresses—heat, cold, lack of oxygen, compression, decompression, acceleration, vibration and noise— have been established. Medicine is bound to be intimately concerned with this new field of applied physiology because the prevention of injury to the actual explorers is clearly a doctor's work. Because national prestige and security rather than the quest for scientific knowledge underlie the research, and because the human volunteers are genuinely willing, the only ethical doubts are in the minds of those who make the experiments. Some may question the use to which the new knowledge is put. No one questions their right to make the experiments. Moreover, the results of this research promise to help people much nearer home. Indeed, as we shall see, they have already done so.

This chapter is concerned, then, with a discussion, inevitably brief, of each of these frontiers; with the disorders man experiences if he crosses them; and with the practical uses to which this new knowledge is being put. With experiments on sensory deprivation, arising again from the needs of war, psychological frontiers are being explored. This research, too, is being turned to use for the man in the street. Lastly in concentration camps a terrible experiment was made, in a clumsy unwitting way, on human tolerance to adverse conditions—it would be natural here to use the word stress, but as already explained in the last chapter this word's meaning in medicine is now confused and it is best avoided.

In this chapter, in brief, the subjects are those diseases and disorders that are either self-imposed or are imposed on others.

Heat

Outsiders who have gone to live in hot climates have learnt from their hosts, who are naturally adapted to them, and from experience. Systematised knowledge of the effects of heat accumulated quickly, however, from the needs of armies fighting in tropical conditions and oilfield explorers. Laboratories in which variables can be controlled have been set up. By now the several syndromes of the heat disorders have been defined—heatstroke, heat syncope, heat cramps, heat exhaustion, etc.—and there is broad international agreement on nomenclature. The importance of acclimatisation, of clothing and of humidity is recognised and methods of prevention and of treatment are well established. Indeed, it is probably the inhabitants of temperate climates caught unprepared by a sudden heat wave who are most likely to suffer from the harmful effects of heat.

A special problem has recently arisen and has led to concentrated research. During the re-entry of a space vehicle into the denser layers of the earth's atmosphere its surface becomes extremely hot. The enormous heat generated on the broad forward surface creates technical problems; in addition, unless insulation is provided, with its penalty of increased weight, the internal surface of the capsule is bound to get very hot indeed. There are two aspects of human tolerance to high air and wall temperatures: heat storage, in which the body behaves rather like a tank of water that slowly takes up heat from its surroundings; and skin temperature. During re-entry heat storage presents few problems for the duration is only about fifteen minutes. If, however, human skin temperature reaches 113°F. (45°C.) severe pain is experienced. Adequate clothing, so long as metal fasteners do not produce a leakage of heat inwards, effectively ensures that the skin temperature does not reach this figure. In fact, in a research oven, a man totally enclosed in a suit ventilated with cold air was able to tolerate an air and wall temperature of 500°F. for more than fifteen minutes.[1]

Heat has its uses in medicine. It is used locally in physiotherapy applied to the skin on the supposition that it increases the blood supply to underlying tissues. At one time it was also employed in the form of hyperthermia in the treatment of general paralysis, a variety of syphilis of the nervous system. Fever was produced, either by infection of the patient with malaria or by confining his body in a heated box. Even if now superseded by penicillin this form of treatment should at least be remembered as the first successful form of physical treatment in psychiatry.

Cold

Again, as with exposure to heat, the body's response to cold has been studied for centuries. The syndromes are well known; preventive methods are established; and many of the consequences can be treated. Wars in cold climates, mountaineering, polar exploration and shipwreck have yielded a wealth of information. On the whole

[1] Webb, P. in *Bioastronautics* ed. Schaefer, K. E. (Macmillan. New York, 1964).

those who live in these climates have learnt how to protect themselves. This is not always the case with those who live in apparently mild climates and who, in their climbing, walking, sailing and pot-holing, underestimate the lethal effects of a combination of cold, wet and wind. In bad conditions the tired, poorly clad and underfed can die from hypothermia even when the external temperature is above freezing point. Dr Pugh has described twenty-three climbing and walking accidents in the last few years in Wales, Scotland, Cumberland and Derbyshire, which led to twenty-five deaths, nearly all in young people.[1][2] He remarks that four of the dead were unusually thin and lacking in subcutaneous fat, a characteristic also of those who have a low resistance to cooling in water. Many were ill-clad and ill-prepared.

Two other groups of people are particularly at risk from the cold— premature babies and the extremely aged. The former have immature heat-regulating systems and, in addition, their body-surface, which determines heat loss, is large in comparison with their bulk, which determines heat production. That accidental hypothermia is a common risk in elderly people and a common cause of death has only been recognised recently.[3] Many reasons, biological and social, contribute to it. Aged people often lose bulk, particularly their subcutaneous fat, so that heat production and insulation fall without much compensatory shrinkage of body surface. In addition their ability to step up heat production in response to exposure to cold becomes sluggish and they may lose the capacity to shiver. Failing mental powers, poverty, isolation, feebleness and other physical handicaps may make them take few precautions to protect themselves. Some drugs, too, the barbiturates and the phenothiazines such as chlorpromazine, which may have been prescribed for sleeplessness or because of confusion, directly affect temperature regulation. Alcohol can be noxious because it increases loss of heat. Once the hypothermic old person is discovered and the condition has been diagnosed admission to hospital is essential. Any belief that treatment by surface rewarming with hot-water bottles, electric blankets and hot baths would be simple and effective should be abandoned. Such methods are in fact dangerous, because by attracting scarce blood to the body surface they rob vital areas, particularly the brain, of their blood supply, and by distributing cold blood from the surface to the internal organs they may provoke a lethal "after-drop" in internal body

[1] Pugh, L. G. C. (1964), *Lancet*, **i,** 1210.
[2] Pugh, L. G. C. E. (1966), *Brit. Med. J.*, **i,** 123.
[3] *Accidental Hypothermia in the Elderly*. A report by a special committee of the B.M.A. (1964), *Brit. Med. J.*, **ii,** 1255.

temperature. The aim is to increase the temperature of the body far more slowly, by not more than 1°F. (0.56°C.) per hour. Even so, hospital treatment can only save perhaps one-third of these old people. Hypothermia can be surprisingly deadly, and prevention is far easier than cure.

Cold has been used as an ally in medicine. At ordinary body temperature if the brain is deprived of blood for about three minutes irreparable damage will be done. Other vital tissues, heart muscle and kidney, for example, can only survive similar short periods of deprivation. At lower temperatures these organs can survive for much longer, the time depending roughly on the drop in temperature. Deliberate cooling of the body has made surgery on the open heart possible. The cooling is achieved gradually either by removing blood continuously from a vein and passing it through a heat exchanger before returning it to an artery, or by general body cooling, or in both ways. In cardiac and arterial surgery, and in neurosurgery, cooling to 86°F. (30°C.) or even as low as 48°F. (9°C.) has been employed and can give the surgeon half-an-hour or perhaps more in which to carry out his work in a bloodless field and on a heart that has stopped beating. Techniques of cooling and rewarming, which belong to anaesthesia, are by now rich in variety and far from simple. They carry, certainly with extreme cooling, much risk to life and health; but so do the diseases and abnormalities that they help to cure—faulty valves in the heart, weaknesses and blockages in arteries, tumours of the brain. But for these techniques many of the developments in cardiac surgery—repair to valves and replacements— would have been impossible. The development of more efficient heart-lung machines, which exclude the heart from the circulation, is tending to mean that hypothermia is less often employed today.

Compression and Decompression

In caissons used in building the foundations of bridges and in the shields used in tunnelling under rivers and marshes men work in compressed air. The high pressure prevents water from entering the workings. If these men return too quickly to normal atmospheric pressure, the excess nitrogen that has been dissolved under pressure in their blood and tissues can form bubbles and cause decompression sickness (Caisson disease, "the bends"). The illness was described over a hundred years ago by Bucquoy,[1] and a liability to suffer from

---

[1] Bucquoy, E. (1861), *Action de l'air comprimé sur l'économie humaine.* M.D. thesis. (University of Strasbourg). Quoted in Miles, S. *Underwater Medicine.* (Staples Press, London, 1962).

it is created whenever the atmospheric pressure falls rapidly. Thus, the diver ascending fast, the man who escapes from a crippled submarine, people in aeroplanes when pressurisation fails, and the astronaut hurled a hundred miles high in a few minutes will all be at risk.

The symptoms vary with the speed and extent of the decompression; those who are mildly affected complain only of aching pain in or near a joint, burning feelings or tingling in the skin, and exhaustion. The more serious cases develop "the chokes" —pain in the chest, severe shortness of breath, rapid pulse, pallor and collapse—or "the staggers"—giddiness, disturbed vision and paralysis.

The condition is much more easily prevented than cured. In the air, failure of pressurisation compels a swift return to lower altitudes because of the even more serious risk of lack of oxygen. Divers and caisson workers have to be recompressed, either by returning to where they came from or else in a decompression chamber if one is available. Recompression relieves the symptoms, and subsequently a slower return to sea-level pressure prevents the same thing from happening again. Astronauts are protected in a number of ways against "the bends" during a rapid climb. According to reports[1] the Russians use ordinary air at sea-level pressure in their space craft. They rely on a pressure suit in case the pressurised cabin should leak. On the other hand the American astronauts breathe pure oxygen at a pressure of 259 mm Hg[2] in the capsule and in their pressure suits. To prevent "the bends" from developing they breathe an atmosphere of pure oxygen for two or three hours before blast-off. In this time most of the nitrogen in their blood and tissues diffuses slowly out. In theory even bubbles of oxygen leaving the tissues under swift decompression could cause symptoms—indeed, in an experiment with goats[3] this has been shown to happen; but so rapidly is oxygen used up in the tissues that these symptoms disappeared completely in five minutes without recompression.

But compression has other dangers apart from those of subsequent decompression. In the last thirty years nitrogen narcosis has been increasingly recognised as a risk to deep sea divers and to others who are breathing air under high pressure. Originally described in 1935 by Captain Behnke[4] in the United States its vulgar name is "the narks".

[1] Schaefer, K. E. in *Bioastronautics*.
[2] Air pressure at sea level = 760 mm. mercury (Hg) = 33 ft. sea water = 14·7 pounds per sq. in. (psi) = 1 atmosphere.
[3] Donald, K. W. (1955), *J. Appl. Physiol.*, **7**, 639.
[4] Behnke, A. R., Thomson, R. M. and Motley, E. P. (1935), *Amer. J. Physiol.*, **112**, 554.

M

Captain Cousteau,[1] however, has produced a more descriptive name
—"l'ivresse des grands profondeurs". He records a colleague's
description of a record dive: ". . . I really feel wonderful. I have a
queer feeling of beatitude. I am drunk and carefree. My ears buzz
and my mouth tastes bitter. The current staggers me as though I had
had too many drinks." Nitrogen narcosis can come on at depths
greater than 100 feet (4 atmospheres); its symptoms range from light-
headedness, euphoria and garrulity to rash unconcern for safety and
ultimately unconsciousness. "If a passing fish seems to require air
the crazed diver may tear out his air pipe or mouth grip as a sublime
gift."[2] Experienced divers can acquire a degree of adaptation to
hyperbaric nitrogen and can tolerate dives to greater depths than
novices.

The consequences of lack of oxygen have long been familiar—the
breathlessness, the blueness, the changes in behaviour. These are the
same whether the anoxia is caused by diseases such as heart failure,
severe anaemia, or pneumonia, by mountaineering above 12,000
feet, or by failure of pressurisation in an aircraft. That oxygen can
also be toxic is a much less familiar idea. But oxygen posioning can
indeed happen either as a result of breathing pure oxygen at
atmospheric pressure or from breathing air under pressure. It seems
to be established that breathing concentrations of oxygen up to 60%
(a partial pressure of 460 mm Hg) can do no harm. Concentrations
above this value and partial pressure of oxygen higher than this level
such as are encountered at a pressure of more than three atmospheres
(66 feet of water) lead in time to oxygen poisoning. If dives are made
while the diver is breathing pure oxygen very high partial pressures
of oxygen are soon encountered. Experiments have shown that within
fifteen minutes at 80 feet down one person in two will develop tremors,
twitchings, giddiness and a feeling of sickness. If the pressure is
maintained convulsions follow, and a sudden convulsion may in fact
be the first sign of oxygen intoxication. In the Royal Navy it is now
customary to limit dives that involve exertion to 25 feet if pure
oxygen is being used.[3] For deeper dives oxygen/nitrogen mixtures
have to be employed.

The use of pure oxygen at atmospheric pressure takes longer—
hours or even days—to produce harmful effects. Many organs may
be affected, but the chief damage is to the lungs. A dry cough and
soreness of the chest are the symptoms that result from the under-

---

[1] Cousteau, J. Y. *The Silent World*. (Hamish Hamilton. London, 1953).
[2] Cousteau, J. Y., ibid.
[3] Miles, S. *Underwater Medicine.*

ying congestion and bronchitis. Jet pilots breathing pure oxygen have sometimes suffered a collapse of part of a lobe of one lung, though this collapse may be partly caused by the pressure suits, which restrict chest expansion. Oxygen-tents have therefore to be used with caution in the treatment of acute and chronic chest conditions.

One special danger of oxygen was recognised in 1952. Many premature babies need oxygen in their first few days of life to alleviate distressed and inefficient breathing. But it has been found that the use of a high concentration of oxygen over long periods in their incubators leads to an increased risk of blindness. Paediatricians, therefore, have to give them a sufficient concentration of oxygen to save their lives but not so much as to cause blindness from retrolental fibroplasia.

The introduction of oxygen under pressure—hyperbaric oxygen— as a treatment for a variety of conditions is therefore not without its risks. The risk of blindness is confined to premature and newborn babies, but there are other risks—fire, for example, ruptured ear drums and oxygen poisoning. Nevertheless, despite the risks, this is an active growing point in medicine and month by month the list of conditions in which hyperbaric oxygen therapy is being used lengthens. For the treatment either a one-man chamber is used, or a pressure chamber big enough to contain the patient, who breathes pure oxygen, and one or more attendants, who breathe air. They, naturally, risk decompression sickness later unless precautions are taken to prevent it.

In the treatment of carbon monoxide poisoning oxygen under pressure corrects the lack of oxygen in the tissues almost at once, and it increases the rate at which the gas is removed from the blood. Coal gas poisoning is still a very common method of suicide in Britain, and though few die once they have reached hospital, a hyperbaric oxygen chamber would certainly save some lives and would limit the extent of brain damage in other patients. Its value in this condition can be regarded as well established.

But there are further ways in which hyperbaric oxygen is proving to be life-saving: in the treatment of gas-gangrene and in radiotherapy for some cancers. Infection with the gas-producing organism *Clostridium welchii* is a rare consequence of wounds and of operative surgery. It has a high mortality once it is established. This organism is anaerobic and flourishes in the absence of oxygen. High-pressure oxygen inhibits its growth and multiplication, arrests the disease, and results in a dramatic improvement in the patient's condition. Professor

Boerema of Amsterdam, who introduced this form of treatment in 1960, reported later[1] on a successful series of 26 patients treated with oxygen in a pressure chamber. Only four died and two of these deaths were unrelated to the gas-gangrene infection—a far better result than has been achieved with other methods of treatment.

The sensitivity of both normal and malignant cells to X-rays is much diminished by lack of oxygen in the fluid surrounding them at the time; it is little, if at all, increased by excessive oxygen. There is firm evidence that a small proportion of the cells in malignant tumours, perhaps 1 %, lack oxygen and that they are only about one third as sensitive to radiation. They may survive therapeutic radiation doses and by their continued multiplication can cause the treatment to fail. The reason for the use of hyperbaric oxygen in radiotherapy, therefore, is not an attempt to make all the cells in a tumour more sensitive, but to try to ensure that there are no anoxic insensitive cells present at the time that the dose of radiation is given. The treatment has now been used for twelve years or more and some impressive results have been reported. One must remember that the technique has largely been confined to patients with advanced disease unsuitable for other forms of treatment. In these circumstances a five year survival rate of 12 % is encouraging.[2]

Other uses to which oxygen under pressure can usefully be applied include skin grafting, chronic infections such as osteomyelitis, and threatened gangrene of part of a limb because of arterial disease or injury. Recently, too, a one-man chamber has been devised, in which the patient can breathe oxygen at two atmospheres while either lying down or sitting-up. At the Westminster Hospital, London, forty patients with severe coronary attacks have been treated for periods of two hours at a time in such a chamber. Many distressing symptoms, pain in particular, were immediately relieved; only three patients died. It is possible that the use of oxygen under pressure may reduce the mortality of severe myocardial infarction treated in hospital from the present 20–30 % to 10 % or less. The initial cost of the machine is high, but the cost per patient might be reduced from the present figure if, as seems likely, the length of stay in hospital is thereby shortened.

Acceleration and Deceleration

In a vacuum, as every schoolboy knows, any object, a pound of lead

[1] Brummelkamp, W. H., Boerema, I. and Hoogendyk, L. (1963), *Lancet*, **i**, 235.
[2] Churchill-Davidson, I. (1964). *Proc. Roy. Soc. Med.*, **57**, 635.

or a pound of feathers, will fall towards the centre of the earth with a velocity that increases by 32·4 feet per second each second. This acceleration caused by gravity is termed g. Accelerations and decelerations due to other forces—rockets, aeroplane engines and collisions—are measured in the same units and termed G. The devastating effect on the human body of high G-forces and high g from sudden arrest after free falls and from collisions have been obvious enough ever since man used weapons, rode horses, or threw themselves off tall buildings. For a long time, too, people have been fascinated by the physiological effects of the mildly raised G-forces and lowered g that they can experience in fair grounds on roller-coasters, on the Whip, swings, the Rotor and in fast lifts. Many of these feelings, sensations of rotation, dizziness, sinking feelings, sensations of the heart rising into the mouth, are common symptoms of anxiety: it is curious that most of mankind will pay money to experience them while the rest visit doctors to be rid of them. Angular velocity produces a centrifugal G-force which, if it is in the plane passing through the centre of the earth, will be an anti-g acceleration and lead to partial or complete weightlessness.

The accelerations reached in high speed aircraft, and even more in the rocket-propelled vehicles that are fired into orbit, have stimulated a huge volume of physiological research into human tolerance of high-G and of zero-g, the weightless state. Although valuable experiments have been made elsewhere in the Western world and must have been made in Russia too, the resources devoted to the subject in the United States, the variety and scale of the technical equipment there, and the amount that has been published make acceleration research very much an American preserve. The following account relies mainly therefore on two American sources.[1] [2] In 1964 the United States possessed five human centrifuges with several more under construction and at least one with a radius of 50 feet; another had been adapted to support a slow rotation room, 15 feet in diameter, in which men could live for days on end while the room rotated at speeds of up to ten revolutions per minute; very rapid linear accelerations and decelerations have been studied in drop-towers or with rocket, ram-jet, or pneumatically powered horizontal and vertical sleds on tracks with powerful frictional or hydraulic braking systems.

Linear acceleration mainly affects the long columns of blood in

[1] *Physics and Medicine of the Atmosphere and Space* ed. Benson, O. O. and Strughold, H. (John Wiley. New York, 1960).
[2] *Bioastronautics*, ed. Schaefer, K. E.

the body and the mobile viscera within the chest and abdomen. If the acceleration is applied in the long axis of the body and towards the head, blood, because of its inertia, will be left behind and will tend to drain from the head into the extremities. The blood pressure at the base of the brain will drop, causing progressively loss of peripheral vision, "grey-out", "black-out" and loss of consciousness. For the average and unprotected man these phenomena occur at accelerations between 4 and 5·5 G—that is, 130–180 feet per second every second. When the direction of acceleration is reversed but is still in the body's long axis, the phenomenon of "red-out" is experienced. This is not caused by an excess of blood in the eye itself but by swelling and upward movement of the lower lids, which rise to cover part of the cornea in a thin layer.

Transversely applied acceleration front-to-back or back-to-front is much better tolerated than longitudinally applied accelerations. At about 8 G there is difficulty in breathing because of the muscular effort involved in lowering the diaphragm and pushing the sternum forwards, and there is pain, too, behind the sternum. Small blood vessels in the skin may rupture.

Tolerance of high-G is greatly improved by partial pressure suits, which prevent viscera from shifting and which diminish pooling of blood either upwards or downwards. The design of seats and couches, particularly the adoption of a semi-supine position on a couch that orientates itself automatically so that the subject faces directly towards the G-force increases tolerance even more. In experiments men have been able to withstand 23 G for up to four seconds and to perform complex tasks for three minutes at 12 G. These accelerations are far in excess of the maxima of 8 G encountered on the upward journey in the American Mercury and Gemini flights and of the 5 G met with in the Saturn programme.

Re-entry into the earth's atmosphere not only creates problems of heat-tolerance for both the vehicle and its occupants but can also easily give rise to G-forces that are far beyond human endurance. A vehicle returning vertically from space could subject its occupants to 300 G. Re-entry therefore has to be made at a shallow angle to bring both the heat and deceleration within acceptable human and structural limits. But re-entry, unlike blast-off, is complicated by two exacerbations of G: the opening of the parachute, which can produce a deceleration of 8 G lasting for 2 seconds; and water impact, which may cause up to 40 G for 0·05 second.

In the foreseeable future, however, few people are going to be subjected to the G-forces of blast-off or re-entry. More, unhappily, will be in aircraft that fly into mountains or hit the ground at high speed, and many more still will be in colliding motor vehicles. For them research into acceleration, or rather deceleration, is very relevant.

The best known research into the tolerance of humans and chimpanzees to high decelerations of very short duration such as are met with in road collisions has been carried out with rocket-powered sledges running on rails.[1][2][3] Decelerations from 120 miles per hour to a stop in 19 feet can be survived by human beings without injury. This is equivalent to a deceleration of 40 G for 0·2 seconds with a rate of onset of 600 G per second. Such stresses can be tolerated only if an efficient harness is worn consisting of a lap strap and chest strap, and if the back-facing seat has a head rest, arm rests with hand holds, leg supports and wings to prevent sideways movement. Such research, undertaken to establish human tolerance to the stresses of space flight, re-entry, and ejection from aircraft at high speed, is obviously capable of adaptation to help minimise the effects of road collisions.

Already, however, acceleration research has proved to be of value in medicine. According to a report from the Mayo Clinic, a human centrifuge has been successfully used in the treatment[4] of a patient with a detachment of the retina. A force of between two and three G was used for more than two hours with the head carefully positioned so as to induce the detached part of the retina to lie back in place. The older technique of thermo-coagulation was then employed to anchor it.

Weightlessness

At the opposite extreme from the high accelerations and decelerations of impacts, take-off into orbital flight, and re-entry is the state of zero-g or weightlessness. Here the pull of gravity is exactly balanced by the centrifugal force generated by the capsule's velocity of almost 18,000 miles per hour. The weightless state can be experienced for less than a minute in high speed aircraft following a parabolic trajectory, and this brief experience has been used in training the crews of spacecraft. But longer experience of weightlessness has had to await successful orbital flight. Many of the effects predicted from theory have either not materialised or have proved easy to tolerate

[1] Stapp, J. P. (1955), *J. Aviation Med.*, **26,** 268.
[2] Stapp, J. P. (1957), *Amer. J. Surg.*, **93,** 734.
[3] Eiband, A. M. *Human Tolerance to Rapidly Applied Acceleration: a summary of the literature.* N.A.S.A. Memorandum. 5-19-59E. (1959).
[4] Neault, R. W., Martens, T. G., Code, C. F. and Nolan, A. C. (1966), *Mayo Clinic Proc.*, **41,** 145.

or surmount; most of the people who have experienced weightlessness have found it positively pleasant and even exhilarating.

Both speculation and such brief experiments as could be done on earth had led to predictions that a number of serious disturbances of physiology would be common in the weightless state:

a. Labyrinthine function: the utricle and saccule of the labyrinth of the inner ear with their otoliths ordinarily give information about linear acceleration and, because of the pull of gravity, about the position of the head in space; the semi-circular canals give information about movements of the head both linear and angular. This information in the normal man in normal conditions is co-ordinated with information from the eyes and about the position of the joints and the stretch on muscles to give a very complete picture of his orientation in space and his linear and circular motion. In the weightless state, the ordinary pull of gravity on the otoliths will be missing; stretch sensations from the body's weight on muscles will be reduced; and, in a capsule, visual clues may be absent. This might be expected to lead to total disorientation, incapacity to perceive the vertical and, because of a conflict of evidence from various sources, to motion sickness, nausea, vomiting, sensations of spinning and loss of co-ordination between hand and eye. In experiments on 46 men and one woman during brief exposure to weightlessness lasting for about half a minute, 14 experienced quite severe motion sickness and a further 11 milder symptoms—slight disorientation, dizziness and nausea. No doubt these experiments and experience on the human centrifuge have screened out those who are particularly liable to physiological disturbance under high or low G-forces. It is not surprising, therefore, that of the first ten human beings, Russian and American, to experience prolonged weightlessness in orbit only one reported any labyrinthine disturbance—a Russian after his sixth orbit, who had sensations resembling sea sickness if he turned his head sharply. These may have been caused in fact not by zero-g but by some abnormal tumbling motion of the capsule.[1]

b. Swallowing and digestion: without gravity, precautions have to be taken to anchor stray objects so that they do not float about in the cabin. This applies especially to fluids because of the danger of inhalation. Food has to be taken therefore largely in the form of fluid or paste sucked or squeezed from a container. Swallowing, however, presents no difficulty. It is dependent not on gravity but on a squeeze-

[1] Shaefer, K. E. *Bioastronautics.*

wave travelling from the pharynx to the stomach. Indeed patients in hospital who have to be nursed with their feet higher than their head find little difficulty in swallowing uphill.

In parabolic jet experiments some people tended to regurgitate stomach contents, but in all the orbital flights there has been no mention of digestive upset of any kind. Nor do any difficulties seem to have been encountered with excretion although the mechanical manoeuvres must be intricate.

c. Circulation and respiration: the rapid pulse and shallow laboured breathing associated with the high-G forces of the launch are succeeded by a rapid return to normal in the weightless state. It has been suggested that prolonged weightlessness, like lying motionless in bed, would lead to general loss of tonus in the cardio-vascular system and to a fall in blood pressure, but in the Russian and American orbital flights there has been as yet no evidence of this happening in flights lasting five days. No doubt, regular exercises during the trip contribute to this immunity to serious circulatory symptoms, such as unconsciousness, during re-entry. This must resemble taking part in a three mile race immediately after a week in bed.

d. Changes in muscle and bone: like the patient confined strictly to bed the astronaut in his weightless state will lose muscle tone and his bones will lose calcium. But this is a slow process, unlikely to develop significantly in under two weeks, and it can be prevented or at least discouraged by regular exercise. In long flights, if mobilisation of calcium from bones cannot be avoided, there could well be a risk of kidney stones forming.

e. Sleep: the unfamiliarity of weightlessness and the haphazard occurrence of day and night could well be expected to interfere with sleep. In fact the experience of those who have been in orbit so far is that sleep is fitful at first but later becomes more normal. It seems helpful to impose an arbitrary rhythm quite independent of the light or dark sky and to exclude light from the capsule for a set period in every twenty-four hours. So far there is no information available from EEG records of astronauts on what proportion of their sleep is orthodox sleep and how much is that paradoxical rapid-eye-movement sleep accompanied by dreams described[1][2][3] by Kleitman in Chicago and by others. If one result of prolonged weightlessness should prove to be deprivation of r.e.m. sleep—though this specula-

[1] Kleitman, N. A. *The Nature of Dreaming.* Ciba Foundation Symposium on the Nature of Sleep. ed. Wolstenholme. (Churchill. London, 1961).
[2] Dement, W. (1963), *Science,* **131,** 1705.
[3] Oswald, I. *Sleeping and Waking.* (Elsevier. Amsterdam and New York, 1962).

tion seems to be unlikely—it could lead to physical deterioration and dangerous falling off in performance of skilled tasks.

f. Performance: in general the earlier experimental work on the efficiency of animals and men under brief conditions of weightlessness has been overtaken by events, and is of little further interest. It is clear that astronauts are able to maintain a high level of skilled performance throughout many days of zero-g. Concentration, accuracy, speed, judgment are unimpaired, so that the pilot of Vostok III was able to say that he did "everything during flight as though he were on the ground".[1] Thus far nothing has been said of the effects on performance of sensory deprivation. The research into this subject is sufficiently important to demand separate discussion later.

The published work on which this account has been based dates from 1964 or earlier. Nothing has happened since then to invalidate the conclusion that weightlessness is a pleasant experience compatible with well-being and efficiency. The longer journeys, the walking in space and the more complex tasks carried out have served to confirm it.

The Vertical Frontier

That man can survive and work in space is no doubt a tribute to his extraordinary adaptability, but even so man's inherent homeostatic mechanisms, which maintain his *milieu intérieur* constant, require a *milieu extérieur* that can only vary physically and chemically within fairly narrow limits. The technical prowess called forth in the exploration of the vertical frontier is a marvel, and an exceptionally costly one, matched only by the courage of those who have entrusted their lives to it. Now that globe-trotting has become almost commonplace we should forget neither the complexity of the technical systems involved in hurling men a hundred miles high, nor the number of factors that have to be controlled in the *milieu extérieur* inside their capsule. Ingenuity has to provide at least the following to avoid discomfort, ill-health and disaster:

an equable temperature; suitable gas for breathing at an appropriate pressure; a means of removing carbon dioxide and water vapour; supplies of food and drink, compact and easily assimilable; means of dealing with excreta, solid, fluid and gaseous; control of G-forces on ascent and re-entry; a curb on noise and vibration; a shield against

[1] Shaefer, K. E. *Bioastronautics.*

:he heat of re-entry; a capsule skin sufficient to resist the impact of
micro-meteorites; means of communication with the earth; ways of
manoeuvring the capsule to stop rotation and tumbling and to
initiate re-entry; equipment for exercising muscles to prevent muscle
and bone atrophy.

If exploration of this frontier is to continue farther on the moon
and beyond, new ranges of problems will need solving if health and
life are to be maintained. Of these the most immediate concern
radiation, for on their way to the moon astronauts will have to
traverse the van Allen radiation belts[1] and while in space they will
be at risk of experiencing sudden increases in the intensity of radiation following solar flares as well as constant background bombard-
ment by cosmic ray particles. Radiation biology is a fast-growing
subject of great complexity, but at present an accurate prediction
of the radiation dosage likely to be received by an astronaut protected
by the skin of his space ship and his clothing is exceptionally difficult.
One informed estimate[2] is that a return trip to the moon would
expose the traveller to perhaps thirteen rads.[3] To put this figure in
context: the recommended upper dosage for people whose work
involves contact with ionising radiations is sixty rads over the total
period between the ages of 18 and 30. The likely dose thus is considerable but not prohibitive; it could be greatly reduced if escape
from the earth's atmosphere in the polar regions proved to be feasible
technically. Unless the occupants of a space ship were unlucky
enough to be travelling at the time of a solar flare they would be
unlikely to suffer to any serious extent from the effects of radiation
either immediately (radiation sickness, vomiting, anaemia, eye
damage, loss of hair, impairment of skilled performance) or later
(leukaemia, genetic damage, accelerated ageing). There is, moreover,
the possibility that less toxic and more effective chemical "pro-
tectors" against radiation than the drug cysteamine might be discovered, so that tolerance could temporarily be increased to cope
with some emergency.

As men are unlikely to get farther in space than the moon for many

[1] Two belts described by J. A. van Allen in 1958 consisting of intensely charged particles,
protons and electrons, trapped in the geomagnetic field. The smaller inner belt extends
from 1,000km to 8,500km above the earth's surface; the outer consisting largely of electrons, extends from 10,000km to 60,000km above the earth. Both, maximal at the equator,
are missing at or near the poles.

[2] Alexander, P. and Rosen, D., in *The Biology of Space Travel.*, ed. Pirie, N. W. Symposia
of the Institute of Biology, No. 10. (London, 1961).

[3] The rad is the unit of absorbed ionising radiation. A single dose of 500 to 1,500 rads is
lethal.

years, and as the problems of longer journeys in space are more technical than medical they hardly need discussion here. One might reasonably expect, however, that as days lengthen into weeks, and as tasks and companions become all too familiar in the cramped quarters of a space-ship, psychological difficulties may become more troublesome than they have been hitherto. Prolonged weightlessness, even if partially counteracted by the artificial gravity of circular motion, might be harmful in these long runs, and the monotony of the diet, especially if food came from some recycling system employing algae—a solution to the weight problem that has struck the imagination—could easily contribute to ill-health, discontent and impaired efficiency and zest. In such conditions the emotional hell forecast by Admiral Byrd[1] for a two-man Antarctic base might come true: "But the time comes when one has nothing left to reveal to the other; when even his unformed thoughts can be anticipated, his pet ideas become a meaningless drool, and the way he blows out a pressure lamp or drops his boots on the floor or eats his food becomes a rasping annoyance . . ." With this remark we have arrived at the psychological frontier.

Sensory Deprivation

There is a number of situations in which modern man finds himself at the limits of his psychological tolerance. Insofar as the elements of these situations can be analysed they consist of combinations of such factors as fear and intense anxiety, social isolation, confinement, detachment, and a reduction of sensory stimulation. Several of these factors are at work, for example, in one man expeditions by boat or beneath the sea; in journeys into space; in caves; in long distance night driving; in radar observation on isolated stations; and in the period of solitary imprisonment that precedes or initiates the technique of brainwashing. By their very nature many of these factors defy scientific observation, for the presence of an observer in itself would nullify them. Nor could any experiment that involved terrorising men be countenanced by scientists. The only information about the effects of several factors of this kind comes, therefore, from first-hand accounts of people's experiences—from introspection, with, for the scientist, all its drawbacks. The exception, sensory deprivation, has provoked a great deal of research in the past twelve years. The results, which define human tolerance to one kind of stress, are of absorbing interest to those whose job it is to make war, to explorers

[1] Byrd, R. E. *Alone*. (Putnam. New York, 1938).

of the uninhabited regions of the earth and of space, and to the ill-intentioned who would unhinge their enemies to make them more compliant. More prosaically they suggest why those who have far to drive at night are wise to listen to a car-radio, and they might even plausibly explain the menacing shadows and bogymen, the terror of some children's nights. All this belongs more to psychology than to medicine, and would concern us little, were it not that the occurrence of hallucinations, of persecutory ideas, and of loss of insight, which can happen in conditions of sensory deprivation, suggests a *prima facie* relationship to schizophrenia.

The experiments have been, broadly speaking, of two types: those in which the aim has been to reduce sensory input to an absolute minimum and to observe what happens to people over a period of many hours in these conditions; those in which experimental subjects are asked to concentrate on intellectually arduous work that includes problem solving, monitoring and perceptual discrimination over long periods in conditions of greatly reduced sensory input. These latter mimic the actual working conditions in aeroplanes, radar posts, spacecraft and road vehicles.

The former type of experiment originated at McGill University in 1954[1] under Professor Hebb. They have continued there and in many other places, notably Princeton,[2] since then. The experimental conditions have varied much in detail: visual stimuli are reduced either by the subject being in total darkness or by his wearing translucent but not transparent glasses; auditory stimuli are reduced to a minimum either by as near perfect soundproofing of the experimental room as possible or by the masking of all extraneous noise by a constant low hum; tactile stimuli are minimised by a couch and pillow of soft foam rubber, by gloves and elbow-to-finger-tip cuffs or even by near-complete immersion in water; rigorous precautions are taken to prevent the need for food and for excretion from interrupting the deprivation more than they have to.

There is great individual variation of response even when the conditions are held as nearly as possible the same; one man may underestimate the passage of time, for example, by thirty hours or more in ninety-six hours whereas others may be accurate to within four hours. As between different laboratories the results can be so conflicting as to suggest that some apparently quite trivial discrepancy in the conditions—efficient blindfolding during an interruption for excretion, for example—may be crucial, so that

[1] Bexton, W. H., Heron, W. and Scott, T. H. (1954), *Canad. J. Psychol.*, **8**, 70.
[2] Vernon, J. A. *Inside the Black Room.* (Souvenir Press. London, 1963).

hallucinations in the one may be as common as they are rare in the other.

In general, if sensory deprivation in these experiments proves to be tolerable at all—and for some it was not though others could bear seven days—the effects can be summarised as follows: there is an initial period of sleep which may occupy most of the first twenty-four hours; later, sleep is difficult and comes in snatches; boredom and hunger for stimuli mount together with suggestibility so that any novelty is welcome and therefore the susceptibility to propaganda enhanced; disorientation in time develops almost always in the direction of underestimating the time that has elapsed; concentration on intellectual tasks is impaired, but paradoxically in some experiments the speed of learning simple tasks such as a word list is improved; visual hallucinations, simple and more complex, develop in a significant proportion of people, together with perceptual distortions and illusions (25 out of 29 subjects at McGill had hallucinations, and other authors have reported similar figures). On the other hand, in the Princeton experiments only 10 out of 55 people became hallucinated. There is a discrepancy here that is not entirely explained by the observation that hallucinations are less common in total darkness than when some unpatterned light filters through translucent goggles. All the investigators agree that auditory and tactile hallucinations are rare.

Similar phenomena—impaired intellectual functions, disorientation in time, bizarre perceptual experiences and visual hallucinations —have also been reported by those doing research into simulated space flight. Thirty-six hours of sensory impoverishment, during which the subjects had to monitor instruments, respond to signals, render reports, and take rest periods at four-hour intervals, led in some cases to aberrations that in actual flight would have been fatal. A brief summary can only do much less than justice to Dr Hauty's vivid verbatim reports[1] on his subjects' experiences. "The instrument panel (black) phased in rhythmically various colours . . . suddenly, the instrument panel began to melt, very slowly at first, progressively faster within a few seconds or minutes, until, finally, my instrument panel was actually perceived to be dripping on the floor . . . the walls about me appeared to be sloping down to a conical bottomless pit . . . I'm seeing shadows that aren't there, I'm sure, and I'm beginning to see gremlins on the face of this work panel . . . I went through some real flying gravity zero there awhile ago . . . the T.V. set—it's turning brown—right in my face—better turn it off in a hurry—it's getting

[1] *Bioastronautics.*, ed. Schaefer, K. E.

hot as hell—what I'm worried about is the thing exploding . . . I see a wooden man made out of two meters . . . I simply at one point suddenly realised that this was a face, not the meter."

Dr Hauty's experiments were in a sense controlled in that his four subjects "had been made well acquainted with the reasons for and nature of the aberrant experiences likely to occur". His four comparable control flights were made "by subjects who were not given prior notice or instructions concerning these experiences". These controls only reported mild aberrant sensory experiences. This raises a topic that has worried other people. How far do the abnormal experiences of subjects of sensory deprivation depend on suggestion, on briefing about what is to be expected, on the rather terrifying apparatus and the strong hint implicit in the presence of a "panic button"? There is one reported experiment[1] which, if confirmed, could cast doubt on many of the conclusions of sensory deprivation research. Ten paid students believed that they were to take part in an experiment on sensory deprivation. They were questioned by a man in a white coat about their medical history and about any liability to fainting and they were told to report any unusual imagery, fantasies, disorientation and hallucinations. It was emphasised that such experiences were not unusual. A supply of drugs labelled "emergency tray" was prominent; they were told to "try to stick it out if you can"; they were asked to sign a release form exonerating the experimenters if any harmful effects should ensue; and a panic button was openly displayed and its use explained. Ten controls had had a much simpler briefing. They were told that they were part of a control group and there were no white coats, emergency trays, medical history-taking or panic buttons. Each individual spent four hours alone but in a well-lighted uninsulated room with food and an optional task. Thus, they were not in conditions of sensory deprivation. They had psychological tests before and after and they were also asked to comment on any unusual experiences.

The results of the battery of psychological tests showed deterioration in the subjects' performance as compared with the controls'. Perceptual aberrations (the walls of the room starting to waver, impressions of movement in stationary objects, multi-coloured spots seen on the walls), difficulty in concentration, spatial disorientation, restlessness, fears and hostility occurred in both groups but were significantly commoner in the subjects than in the controls.

The authors conclude that the results of many psychological experiments are liable to be biased by those clues, both implicit and

[1] Orne, M. T. and Scheibe, K. E. (1964), *J. Abn. Soc. Psychol.*, **68**, 3.

explicit, that tell the subject what is to be expected in the experimental situation. Clearly this kind of work needs to be repeated on a larger number of people, for to a layman many of the differences that emerged between the heavily briefed subjects and their controls are not very convincing. But one is certainly justified in concluding that the influence of suggestion, the placebo (or rather "monebo") effect, has been neglected for too long in sensory deprivation research. This is not to suggest that the level of sensory input is unimportant—there is too much evidence that it is—but only that at present it is quite uncertain how much of the symptomatology is caused by the "set" of a subject's mind, his fears and expectations.

The results of two other relevant experiments do nothing to resolve these doubts; in fact they raise more. All who have worked in this field state that the effects of sensory deprivation are only experienced in a majority of people after some hours or even days. In 1962 two American psychologists[1] paid fourteen college students to undergo pre-testing, then one hour's sensory deprivation under the usual conditions—translucent goggles, soft couch, earphones with white noise, gloves and cuffs—followed by an interview about their experiences. In the preliminary briefing the students were told about previous peoples' experiences and they were also given innocuous pills but told that the pills were hallucinogenic. Within the hour *all* of them reported a wide variety of unusual experiences—seeing colours and shapes, auditory hallucinations, sensations of bodily movement, feelings of anxiety or of being abandoned, difficulty in thinking, discrepancies in the estimation of time. Many seemed to be convinced of the reality of their experiences and one man had to escape from the room. Suggestion? No doubt, but what of a much earlier experiment reported in 1951 before research on sensory deprivation had even begun?[2] In this there was no question of expectation, briefing, "set" or panic buttons. It was conducted to test the theory that the sensation of colour experienced in a uniform formless but coloured field soon fades to neutral gray. Eleven subjects viewed a uniform red or green field through halves of ping-pong balls fixed over their eyes. The colour did disappear within six minutes, but the authors noted that five of the subjects saw hallucinatory shapes and that this was a threatening and fearful experience.

The relevance of sensory deprivation research to medicine lies in the resemblance between some of the apparent effects of this experience and some schizophrenic symptoms. But the similarities are

[1] Jackson, C. W. and Kelly, E. L. (1962), *Science*, **135**, 211.
[2] Hochberg, J., Triebel, W., and Seaman, G. (1951), *J. Exptl. Psychol.*, **41**, 153.

at best superficial, and it seems highly unlikely that this research will throw much light on the still baffling problems of the cause of schizophrenia. Taken one by one the symptoms of sensory deprivation are seldom the prominent symptoms of a schizophrenic; *in toto* the condition resembles rather an organic psychosis, a mild delirium such as can be caused by alcohol and other toxins, with impaired concentration, mild confusion, disorientation in time, visual illusions and hallucinations, fear, and loss of insight with some secondary paranoid delusions. The hallmarks of the schizophrenic—disordered thinking of a special kind, blunting of emotion, primary delusions, auditory hallucinations and so forth—do not seem to occur. Sleep, except in the early stages of sensory deprivation, is difficult and fitful whereas most schizophrenics sleep very well.

Dr Robert Lifton in his book on brainwashing in China[1] has suggested a further relationship between sensory deprivation and chronic schizophrenia. He draws an analogy between a "deprived milieu" and the chronic wards of old-fashioned mental hospitals in which "patients sat about aimlessly, with little or no challenge or activity-evoking stimuli from their external surroundings". He implies that the milieu causes the illness or at least encourages it to continue. Though every doctor nowadays would agree that such surroundings are harmful and that they are partly responsible for the symptoms of "institutionalisation" if not of schizophrenia no one could pretend that the lack of stimulus in such a ward even remotely resembles the conditions of sensory deprivation experiments described in this chapter.

One further phenomenon concerns medicine. It tends, also, to lend support to those who believe that the consequences of sensory deprivation are due to deprivation and not wholly to suggestion. After an operation on an eye for the removal of a cataract it is the practice to bandage both eyes to exclude light completely and to ensure that the injured eye's repose and recuperation are not jeopardised by movements of the other eye. It is a common experience for some such patients to experience hallucinations during the few days during which light is excluded, and the experience can be upsetting to the extent of inducing a few of them to tear off their bandages.

Practical use of this research is obvious. In space flight, in aeroplanes, and in night driving it is clear that the level of stimulation should be reasonably high and that information should, if possible, be transmitted through more than one sense. Monotony of illumination and of background noise should be avoided and one or more

---

[1] Lifton, R. J. *Thought Reform and the Psychology of Totalism.* (Gollancz. London, 1961)

N

companions would help more by their presence than they would hinder by distracting the pilot in his concentration. For war these techniques could be used to identify those people who would be most likely to break down in conditions of solitary confinement and to train others in ways of resisting brainwashing. As yet there are few indications that research in sensory deprivation has much to offer medicine, but there is one hint in Dr Vernon's book[1] of a possible use which does not yet seem to have been followed up. The two-thirds of his experimental subjects who were smokers found no difficulty whatever in abstaining during their confinement. To a man they said that they seldom thought of the subject during their ninety-six hour sessions and none had any craving. They all, however, returned to the habit on being released. Perhaps a spell inside the black room could help those who seriously want to give up smoking over those first, worst, few days.

If one assumes that, taken together, the evidence from solitary expeditions, from personal experience of solitary confinement, from cataract operations and from experiments is valid, what light does it throw on mental functioning? This question belongs to the realm of pure psychology, and so far no very convincing hypothesis has been suggested which is able to accommodate all the facts. At the least the phenomena of stimulus-hunger and the initial period of sleep, which develop when sensory input is reduced to a minimum, fit in best with, at the neural level, cybernetic theory, and in psychological terms with Gestalt theory. Our perceptual function is organised primarily to extract meaning and significance from the wealth of ordinary sensory input. We search for meaning and, if the input of signals from which it can be sought is limited in the extreme, we extract it still even if the clues are too tenuous to be reliable guides. If necessary, if the clues from the surroundings are too few, we project false clues arising from the brain's own haphazard activity against this flat background and derive false meaning from them. Stimulus-hunger had better be renamed meaning-craving. This more accurately describes one of the most fundamental attributes of mind.

Concentration Camps

No account of the physiological and psychological frontiers, of human tolerance to stresses of one kind and another, could end without an attempt to draw some conclusions from what happened in concentration camps. Here men and women were systematically

[1] Vernon, J. A. *Inside the Black Room.*

destroyed, if not at once in the gas chambers or by being shot, then more gradually like engines being run to destruction. It is sad that from the vastness of the tragedy there is so little to learn: the human tolerance to starvation, to exhaustion, to cold in unprotected surroundings, and to the diseases that flourish in such conditions were already well known; so were the depths of villainy to which ordinary people can plunge under the twin influences of group pressure and evil leadership—the atrocities of war, massacres, pogroms and lynchings have been with us a long time and only the scale and duration are astounding. Familiar, too, are the prodigies of endurance that man is capable of if he feels a renewed hope and that relief is near—as in those last few days at Belsen when diseased, exhausted, emaciated people, near death themselves, were dragging corpses for burial, stumbling, for hours every day, without food or drink, but within sound of British guns.[1]

Nevertheless a great deal has been written on many aspects of concentration camp life—one book lists 150 references.[2] These include descriptions of the physical sufferings and hardships, the behaviour of the inmates, the psychology of the S.S. guards and the infamous and futile medical experiments that went on in these camps. From this wealth of material one can select a few topics for comment either because they are of direct interest to medicine or as shedding light on the human capacity to tolerate the extremes of mental and physical stress: for example, the stages of adaptation to camp life; suicide; the prevalence of some diseases and the rarity of others; and the long-term effects of the concentration camp experience.

In his summary Dr Cohen, who in the course of his imprisonment spent sixteen months late in the war at Auschwitz and three months at Mauthausen, says:

"The human power of adaptation, both mental and physical, is very great, at least much greater than I would have thought possible . . . I would never have thought that a man who was given very inadequate nourishment, who was insufficiently clothed, who slept little, who lived in the worst possible hygienic circumstances and moreover was exposed to all conditions of weather, would still be able to perform heavy physical labour . . . I would not have believed that I could bear the hardships of the death march by the end of January, 1945. I did bear them, and not only did I survive, but I did not even

[1] Le Druillenec, H. O. in *The Trial of Joseph Kramer and Forty-four others*. (The Belsen Trial). ed. Phillips, R. (Hodge. Edinburgh, 1949).
[2] Cohen, E. A. *Human Behaviour in the Concentration Camp*. (Jonathan Cape. London, 1954).

fall ill . . . Who could have imagined that a man on learning that all those who were dear to him had been basely gassed, or on beholding and suffering the atrocities of a concentration camp, would 'merely' respond in the way described in these pages. Would not everyone have expected that a man would have either become acutely psychotic or been driven to suicide?"[1]

Indeed, it is astonishing that the death rate in old-established prisoners fell to 10% per year in these camps. In newer prisoners it was much higher. According to Professor Bettelheim[2] it was as high as 15% a month in the first few months of camp life. These authors agree that only those prisoners capable of adaptation, and among them only the lucky ones, survived; the rest died or were shot. This is a circular definition, of course, valueless unless the peculiar nature of the adaptation is defined. Only in physical terms does the word bear its ordinary meaning; they had to be strong, resistant to disease, capable of hard work on a grossly deficient diet and impervious to a harsh climate against which they had little protection.

The psychological adjustment necessary to survival was far more devious and subtle, demanding qualities not ordinarily regarded as essential to survival. Naturally, those who reacted to their experiences by becoming near-stuporose or by prolonged grief and mourning failed to survive. But equally the combative, the assertive and those who were incapable of submerging their individuality died. They failed to obey the first law of camp life—to be anonymous and unobtrusive—and were shot. By and large, apart from luck, those who survived were people who had some expectation of the appalling things that would happen on the journey or initially at the camp— the physical brutality and the degrading humiliation. Too many arrived in apparently complete ignorance of what went on. Acute depersonalisation, a subject-object split into an I who observes and a me to whom dreadful things were happening, was protective. This was succeeded by a period of mourning, of under-reaction, which, if too severe or prolonged, like stupor and panic reactions was fatal. A "healthy" adaptation compelled a change of values. The prisoner had to live in a world in which he was never alone, in which hunger was an overpowering preoccupation, individuality a mortal crime, and from which compassion and altruism had been all but banished. "The hunger drive is completely overpowering sparing nothing and no one . . . theft, egotism, lack of consideration for others,

[1] Cohen, E. A., op. cit.
[2] Bettelheim, B. *The Informed Heart*. (Thames and Hudson. London, 1954).

pitilessness . . . inside the concentration camp . . . was normal.'[1] The only limit was the risk of being expelled from the prisoner's community. If this happened it was lethal. The surrender of individuality and the all-pervading influence of hunger were paralleled by other regressive changes besides decivilisation: preoccupation with excretory functions, cruelty to new prisoners, childish jealousy, and child-like dependence on authority figures—the S.S. and the prisoners who were in charge of blocks. Ultimately, if he survived, the prisoner became an "old number" resigned to life in the camp. To a greater or lesser extent he had taken on an identification with the S.S., their ideals and values. Life outside the camp had ceased to have much meaning or to hold much interest, and he was mainly concerned with how to live as well as possible within the camp community. A few even dreaded release. Only a minority of prisoners were able ultimately to resist brutalisation. As Dr Meerloo[2] remarks in his dissection of the techniques of brain-washing:

"Tortured and torturer gradually form a peculiar community in which the one influences the other . . . unwittingly he may take over all the enemy's norms, evaluations and attitudes to life. We saw it happen in Germany. The very victims of Nazism came to accept the idea of concentration camps."

Those who survived best in the psychological sense with their personalities, moral outlook and values least eroded were predominantly men and women who were able to retain an inner inviolable preserve beneath all the outward-seeming compromises and conformity to a debased and degraded society. To quote Professor Bettelheim[3] again:

"One had first and foremost to remain informed and aware of what made up one's personal point of no return, the point beyond which one would never, under any circumstances, give in to the oppressor, even if it meant risking and losing one's life."

The possession of a burning faith, political or religious, was protective. Doctors were lucky, not only because in most cases they worked in the somewhat sheltered quarters of the prisoners' hospital but also because their training in scientific observation made a partially detached view possible. They could be viewers as well as participants,

---

[1] Cohen, E. A., op. cit.
[2] Meerloo, J. A. M. *Mental Seduction and Menticide*. (Jonathan Cape. London, 1957).
[3] Bettelheim, B., op. cit.

and though they could not record what they saw they could systematically commit it to memory.

Suicide was quite unusual. During his sixteen months in Auschwitz, Dr Cohen only came to know of one suicide, and he quotes other authors who confirm that suicide was rare in the camps. He says, "the thought of suicide did not occur to me for a single moment". Professor Bettelheim refers to several suicides on the journey to the camp and on arrival, but there seems to be very little doubt that, with the exception of one or two outbreaks of mass suicide, individual suicide was most uncommon in concentration camps. Not even the prisoners who formed the gassing squads at extermination camps committed suicide. They did not do so although they knew that in a few weeks they would be exterminated by a new *Sonder-kommando* as they themselves had gassed their predecessors. Why was suicide so uncommon? In a sense by co-operating in their own extermination many prisoners were passively taking part in a suicidal event and no doubt, too, there may have been an element of suicidal intent in those who succumbed to disease and starvation without a fight. But these deaths lacked the quality of deliberate personal decision that the word ordinarily carries. It was this very quality of personal choice which made the S.S. punish an attempt at suicide severely. Prisoners were not allowed choices. It may well be that the process of adaptation to camp life effectively removed the power to choose. Dr Cohen and other authors have discussed additional possible causes—the absence of elderly people, the familiarity with death in these camps that removed from it any element of fear or reverence. The most plausible view, however, is based on Freud's contention that the suicidal act always contains an element of aggression, a need to punish others and to make them feel guilty. Many prisoners had after some time identified themselves with the S.S. at least partially, and all knew that it was out of the question for any successful suicide to make anybody feel ashamed, guilty or even sorry. The supreme act therefore would be quite pointless.

Overcrowding and lack of time for washing, a deplorable water supply and severe malnutrition—a public health doctor's nightmare —meant that infections of all kinds were rife. It is indeed surprising that the S.S. did not insist on better conditions as a measure of self-protection. Skin infections, gastro-intestinal infection and in particular pulmonary tuberculosis flourished. On liberation from various camps up to 50% of the survivors suffered from active tuberculosis. Severe chronic malnutrition was commonplace especially later on in the war—the *muselmänner*, the walking corpses. "The overwhelming majority were walking skeletons, aged and hideous, keeping on their feet as though by a miracle."[1] Once they had reached this state they had given up the struggle, no longer strove for food, and death was near. Even those who did not succumb lost 30–40% of their body weight. Yet distinct vitamin-deficiency syndromes such as beri-beri, scurvy and pellagra were very uncommon and this slow starvation was almost symptomless apart from famine oedema, which heralded the end.

In contrast to starvation and these infections, many other diseases were conspicuously rare. Diabetes, hypertension, gastric and duodenal ulcers, asthma and eczema, all common enough in civilised communities, were seldom seen. That these illnesses which are often suspected of being psychosomatic, of having a prominent emotional component in their causation, were so rare is perplexing. One could expect that if they were psychosomatic, under conditions of exceptional stress they would have been more rather than less common. Or, are the stresses causing them more specific, conflicts involving self-esteem, self-assertion, hidden hostility, insecurity—conflicts which were overwhelmed by a straightforward necessity to turn all mental energy towards self-preservation and bare survival? Or did selection operate? Were those who were liable to develop psychosomatic complaints eliminated by their incapacity to make the initial adjustment on the transport or in the first week? There seem to be no certain answers.

Deaths in concentration camps did not cease dramatically with liberation. The walking corpses did not automatically revive when given nourishment. Estimates vary of the number of prisoners found alive at Belsen on 15 April, 1945. Figures of 40,000[2] and 60,000[3] have been given. Of these about 13,000 died and not until three weeks later did the number of deaths fall below 200 daily.

Even the survivors had higher death rates than ordinary people of the same age. This finding is in keeping with American reports on the survival of prisoners from Japanese camps.[4] Six years after liberation the total number of deaths was found to have been twice the number to be expected in a group of people of similar age who had not been imprisoned.

It is the long-term psychiatric effects, however, which have aroused

[1] Lingens-Reiner, E. *Prisoners of Fear.* (London, 1948).
[2] Letherby-Tidy, H. and Browne-Kutschbach, J. M. *Interallied Conferences on War Medicine.* (New York, 1947).
[3] Kolb, E. *Bergen-Belsen.* (Verl. f. Literatur. u. Zeitgeschehen. Hanover, 1962).
[4] Wolf, H. G. in *Stress and Psychiatric Disorder.* (Tannes, I. M. 1960).

most interest. Dr Eitinger,[1] for example, between 1957 and 1962 studied various groups of people in Norway and in Israel who had spent long periods in the camps. Some of these were patients in hospitals, others had been referred for examination because of difficulties in readjustment or were attending clinics as out-patients because of nervous symptoms. In each country a third group, which served roughly as a control, was gathered consisting of people who had been fully employed since release and who regarded themselves as healthy. Altogether 590 people were examined. The Norwegian controls, who had in general been exposed to only moderate stress, had escaped serious damage to their personalities. More than a quarter of them, however, had minor nervous symptoms or found that they were especially sensitive and could not bear reading or talking about the war. Of the Israeli controls fewer than 10% were free of symptoms on enquiry. The remainder suffered to a mild degree from what Dr Eitinger calls the concentration camp syndrome, and this in more serious degree characterised the other groups, both Israeli and Norwegian. Fatigue, difficulty in concentration, disturbed sleep, bitterness, irritability, lack of initiative, vertigo, headaches and chronic anxiety were the chief symptoms. The severity of this syndrome was related both to the degree and duration of psychic stress and to the severity of physical damage from head injury, infection with typhus and prolonged malnutrition and weight loss. Even well-integrated people suffered permanent damage, which time did not heal. Irrespective of physical factors this author concludes that psychic trauma can do irreparable harm—at least if it is severe enough: "while the individual was subjected to a brutal and slow form of 'execution', his family was killed, his background torn up, his environment annihilated and his world laid in ruins". Of the schizophrenic and some other psychotic patients he studied he found that in at least half the major causes was their concentration camp experiences. These results have been broadly confirmed by others. In the light of these findings, psychiatrists will have to abandon or modify two cherished beliefs: that psychosis is virtually independent of environmental stress; that the "good personality" does not break under extreme stress, and that, if he does, recovery is quick and complete once the stress has passed.

[1] Eitinger, L. *Concentration Camp Survivors in Norway and Israel.* (Allen and Unwin. London, 1965).

CHAPTER TEN

New Diseases

From Dearth to Plenty

The conditions of life in a concentration camp can serve as a model of a deprived society—starvation, the necessity for hard physical work, the ever-present risk of physical injury and, on the psychological plane, the subjection of all other needs to the will to survive. Conflict with other drives, such as sex and self-esteem, and conflict with conscience were at a minimum. The free expression of the urge to get food to survive was obstructed only by the simple prohibitions of the prisoners' society—in essence "organise what you will from the Germans, but if you steal food from a fellow prisoner you will die". To a lesser extent these conditions in their simplicity were characteristic of the life of most people in "advanced" societies until this century and of life in "underdeveloped" countries still.

The diseases that were common were infections and infestations, pulmonary tuberculosis and deficiency diseases; those that were rare were diabetes, hypertension and arterial disease, gastric and duodenal ulcers, asthma and eczema, and the neuroses. Suicide, too, was seldom even attempted.

The diseases of deprivation have greatly diminished in rich societies as much because of social changes as because of the advances in preventive and therapeutic medicine described in earlier chapters. But those very diseases that were uncommon in concentration camps now plague us instead—arterial disease, diabetes, neurotic and psychosomatic disorders, and an epidemic of attempted suicide which, if not a disease, at least needs treatment and an attempt to prevent its recurrence. Why? Is there any evidence that these and other current afflictions, dental caries, accidents on the road and in the home, alcoholism and drug addiction, cancer of the lung and chronic bronchitis, are caused by lack of "deprivation"? Do an excess of food, a predominantly sedentary existence, and lack of an overwhelming primary drive play any part in causing them? The answers are all

probably "Yes", and to examine them properly would take us deep
into sociology and psychology. Nevertheless these illnesses are coming
more to the fore in medicine; some are increasing in prevalence so
fast as to justify the use of the word epidemic—for example, drug
addiction in the young in Britain and Sweden; others are forcing
medicine to forge new weapons to battle with them—arterial surgery,
alcoholic and addiction units, anti-smoking clinics, and accident
departments. Doctors are being compelled to look beyond the immediate problem, the broken leg of a teenage motorcyclist or an
unconscious woman with aspirin overdosage, to the prior causes in
the individual's personality and situation and, further, to causes in
society itself.

This is not to say that physicians can do very much about these
deeper causes, but at least they can help in trying to identify them
so that those who mould opinion and direct policy are aware of them.
It is plain that the search for prior causes for an event such as a
suicidal attempt becomes more difficult as it extends backwards in
time. Fairly close and verifiable circumstances—poor housing, a
neglectful husband, physical ill health—give way to vaguer concepts
such as inadequacy of personality and a broken-home situation in
childhood. Soon all crispness is lost in a mist of sociological theory
and generalisation. The event is seen to be caused as much by the
setting as by the actor; indeed more, for the setting has to some
extent determined the actor's personality and character.

Theories of personality development are excelled in variety and
mutual exclusiveness only by theories of social pathology. Their
richness can best be expressed in a series of clichés: decline in religious
faith; status seeking; generation gap; search for identity; rootlessness;
rat-race; human condition; uncertainty of role; materialist society;
teenage affluence; belonging; and, of course, keeping up with the
Joneses. These twelve phrases serve to recall theories that have been
held to account for many of the ills of Western society and, by
extension, for many of the illnesses to be discussed in this chapter. No
doubt none will stand up to rigorous analysis any more than did
Lady Wootton's twelve chosen hypotheses of the causes of delinquency in these societies that she dissected so mercilessly a decade
ago.[1]

Yet the theories of medical science, quite inadequate alone as we
have seen to account for many of the illnesses of the old and for many
neuroses, are even less able to accommodate much of the disease to

[1] Wootton, B. *Social Science and Social Pathology*. (George Allen and Unwin. London,
1959). Chap. 3.

be encountered in this chapter. Why, for example, do people start to smoke? Why did that doctor of fifty-five, previously content with a Ford, buy the Ferrari in which he was killed? Why do male university students kill themselves twice, and Oxford and Cambridge undergraduates even more times, as often as men of the same age who are not at a university? Why is the social class distribution of young addicts to hard drugs quite different in England from the United States?

There are no clear answers to these questions in sight. Psychology and social science will have to develop much further before they can provide them. Social medicine, increasingly in the last few decades, has to contend with the sick people concerned although no one knows the causes of their illnesses; but traditional medicine itself has no reason to feel superior, for even there, where "hard" facts are easier to come by, doctors are similarly confused in explaining, for example, diabetes and hypertension. A multifactorial aetiology seems necessary with both proximate and distant elements. Prevention cannot, however, be expected to be very successful until the underlying causes in society and in individual personalities are more accurately defined; and prevention, were the causes known, would be far simpler than treatment, particularly where the "disease" is an addiction or the result of one.

Although it is not possible, because we are so ignorant, to discuss the basic causes of these diseases which are so prevalent in advanced societies, there are points worth considering briefly about many of them. Neurotic and psychosomatic complaints have been mentioned in earlier chapters and will not therefore be discussed again.

Arterial Disease

In some form or other and in one or another site this is responsible for a majority of all deaths in advanced societies. In spite of difficulties and disagreements about terminology and classification, certain facts stand out. Everyone has to die of something and as some causes of death in younger people, such as tuberculosis and other infections, become less common the degenerations of old age claim a larger number of victims. That is one reason why this disease is so common in affluent societies.

Nevertheless diseases of the coronary arteries of the heart cause 30% of deaths in middle-aged men in England and Wales and death rates in this age group have increased by about 40% in the last decade. In younger men, aged 40–44, death from this cause is not now uncommon (0.89 per 1,000 living in 1965) and in this group, and in those even younger, deaths and death rates are increasing faster than in older people[1] (see chart V). The increase in coronary deaths is not confined to Britain and to the United States, where 500,000 deaths from coronary attacks occur each year, but is common

Deaths from heart disease involving the coronary arteries   Chart V

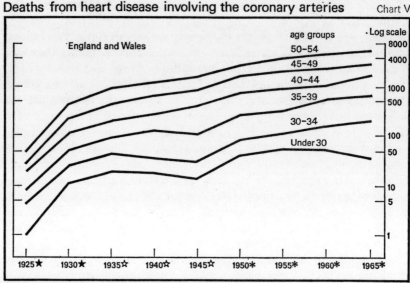

Source: Registrar General's Statistical Reviews. Part I table 17
★ No heading for coronary artery disease. Deaths are included under angina pectoris (94)
☆ Includes angina pectoris (94 b)   ∗ Includes angina pectoris (I.C.D 420·2)

to all countries of Western Europe and to advanced countries elsewhere.

The problem of causes is bedevilled by a confusion between what causes the underlying arterial disease (atheroma), which proceeds either slowly or fast from a beginning often in childhood or adolescence, and what causes symptoms and a sudden thrombotic event. To the evidence that in Western countries death from coronary attacks is becoming commoner in middle age and before can be added evidence that the underlying arterial disease—atheroma—is increasing as well. In Sweden, the United States and Britain comparisons between routine postmortem examinations of those dying of other diseases, of infections and of accidents, carried out in the thirties and in the fifties in this century have shown unmistakable

[1] Oliver, M. F. and Stuart-Harris, C. H. (1965), *Brit. Med. J.*, **ii**, 1203.

evidence of an increase in arterial disease at all ages. Young Americans, too, killed in Korea had a surprising amount of atheroma of their arteries.[1]

At a symposium in Athens in 1966 Dr Howard,[2] in describing the person *least* likely to develop atherosclerosis, is reported to have described her as:

"a hypotensive, bicycling, unemployed, hypo-ß-lipoproteinic, hypolipaemic, underweight, premenopausal female dwarf living in a crowded room on the island of Crete before 1925, and subsisting on a diet of uncoated cereals, safflower oil, and water".

He could also, had he wished, have reasonably described her equally non-atheromatous consort—an ectomorphic Bantu, who works as a London bus conductor, spent the war in a Norwegian prison camp, never eats refined sugar, never drinks coffee and always eats five or more small meals a day. He is taking vast doses of oestrogens to check the growth of his cancer of the prostate.

All these phrases mark correlations established in the last few years in a field of medical research which, in volume at least, is unsurpassed. The conflict of evidence is unequalled as well. "Stress", too, has been implicated—that diffuse and awkward word.[3] To say that a successful, well fed, happily married businessman, whose ultimate ambition is being thwarted by his boss, is suffering from stress, whereas a concentration camp victim or an impoverished peasant is not, is a denial of common sense. Emotional conflict would be a better phrase. Yet even this is inadequate as a description of the tangle of conflicting impulses, emotions and frustrations which affluent man is heir to and which make chronic tension and anxiety such a frequent complaint.

The upshot of all this research into the causes of arterial disease is, so far, highly disappointing. There is much evidence that many factors could be causes; there is so far no evidence of a single preponderant cause; the likelihood at present is that there are several interlocking factors responsible, of which the three most important are overeating, lack of exercise and cigarette smoking—two old vices and one new. Of these some favour the dietary theory, especially as concerns animal fat; others believe that it is quite plausible to pick on

[1] Spain, D. M. *Scientific American.* (August, 1966).
[2] Howard, A. N. *International Medical Tribune of Great Britain.* (30 June, 1966).
[3] The word is used here in its non-extensive, non-Selyean sense to mean only emotional stress.

lack of exercise as perhaps the most important. Professor Morris and his colleagues[1] have shown that for men in the age-range 45–54 during 1949 to 1953 the social class difference in mortality from coronary disease disappears if the degree of physical activity in their work is taken into account. Sedentary workers in social class v had the same high mortality as people in class i. It remains to be seen whether more up-to-date figures will confirm this.

Professor Morris is responsible, too, for a convincing demonstration that the two best indicators of those who are most likely later to have a coronary attack are the blood pressure and the level of cholesterol in the blood plasma. He and his team[2] examined 687 London bus drivers and conductors between 1956 and 1960 and again about five years later. In the interval 47 of them developed evidence of ischaemic heart disease. The incidence was "higher in later than in early middle age, in men with a bad family history of parental death, in drivers than conductors, in cigarette smokers, in the more obese, and in the shortest men". Three quarters of the cases were found in those who, at the earlier examination, were in the top quarter of the group in respect of either systolic blood pressure or blood cholesterol level. These "top-quartiles" have a risk of developing the disease several times as high as the remainder.

These two indicators could certainly serve with others, such as heavy smoking, to screen populations and to identify those at risk. But there would be little point in such an expensive procedure until it becomes clearer that a reduction of blood pressure (by drug treatment) and of blood cholesterol (by restricting the amount of animal fat in the diet) in the symptomless has any preventive value. Hypotensive drugs have unpleasant side-effects and diets designed to lower cholesterol in the blood can be disagreeable; it is too early yet to condemn large numbers of men to a regime of this kind unless the evidence becomes clearer than it is at present. Perhaps the large-scale prospective dietary studies that are now going on in the United States will soon produce a firm answer. Until then the best that the stout middleaged man can do is to eat less, especially less at one sitting, smoke fewer cigarettes, and take more exercise—drab enough advice in all conscience, worthy and simple. Most people would probably prefer something more positive and dramatic such as taking a pill and measuring their own blood pressure daily or even drinking linseed oil before breakfast.

[1] Arie, T. *New Society*, (27 January, 1966).
[2] Morris, J. N., Kagan, A., Pattison, D. C., Gardner, M. J. and Raffle, P. A. B. (1966), *Lancet*, ii, 553.

Cancer of the Lung

At least we now know the predominant cause of this condition in men and we know how to prevent it; yet the epidemic continues. Deaths from this disease in England and Wales in 1935 were 3,598. Thirty years later they were nearly seven times as many and they have doubled since 1950 when in their classical paper[1] Dr Doll and Professor Bradford Hill clearly showed that cancer of the lung and heavy cigarette smoking were closely associated. There is little point in chewing over the evidence, now regarded by almost all people as conclusive, that has subsequently accumulated to show that this cancer is not only associated with heavy cigarette smoking but is also in the main caused by it. Nor is there much to be gained by recalling the wriggling of smokers and of those who peddle tobacco and pander to the addiction in a desperate effort to escape the conclusion, a first triumph for the science of medical statistics, that would rob them of their pleasure and their profit. The manufacturers need not have worried, for while some prudently diversified their production, others no doubt reflected on the strength of tobacco addiction and recalled that prisoners of the Germans on release, and even before their hunger was more than half-satisfied, were seeking, beseeching and looting cigarettes[2] and that for a time after the war these became an unofficial currency in Europe and are still one in prisons.

It is well-known that each year between five and six times as many men as women die from lung cancer. Professor Burn[3] relates this disparity not to any special immunity of women, such as hormonal protection, but to a sex difference in the proportion of smokers who smoke heavily. By marrying the Registrar General's figures for deaths with the Tobacco Manufacturers' Standing Committee's figures of the percentage of smokers who smoke various numbers of cigarettes daily he is able to show that, irrespective of sex, about one person in 115 who smokes more than twenty cigarettes a day will die of lung cancer each year. The risk of death is lower in the young and at a maximum in the age-group 60–69.

This epidemic of lung cancer is common to many of the countries of Europe and North America, and in several of them mortality rates have doubled in a decade.[4] Any direct comparison between countries —for example 89·5/100,000 for males in England and Wales in 1962 (increased to 95·7 by 1965) as against 32·8 for Australia and 23·4 for

[1] Doll, W. R. and Hill, A. B. (1950), *Brit. Med. J.*, **ii**, 739.
[2] Roosenburg, H. *The Walls Came Tumbling Down.* (Secker and Warburg. London, 1957).
[3] Burn, H. *Our Most Interesting Diseases.* (George Allen and Unwin. London, 1964).
[4] WHO. *Epidemiological and Vital Statistics Report.* 1965, vol. 18. no. 7. (Geneva).

Sweden—can mean little unless the age distribution of the population is taken into account. It is the increase within a country that is so significant. Although the death rate in the United States was only 23·1/100,000 population in 1963 this rate was 60% higher than ten years earlier.

One consequence of heavy smoking, even if its role in causing the epidemic of arterial disease is for the moment ignored, has been to

Deaths from pulmonary tuberculosis and lung cancer since 1925 Chart VI

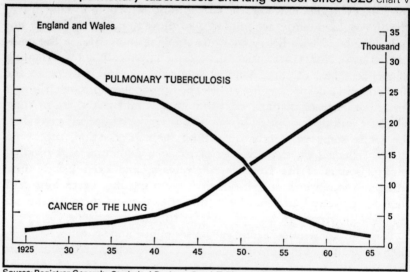

Source: Registrar General's Statistical Reviews. Part I. Tables, medical. Table 7 I.C.D. numbers 002 and 162,163.

throw away, in crude terms, all the lives saved by the hard-earned conquest of pulmonary tuberculosis (see Chart VI).

Once again preventive medicine can succeed only by trying to influence social customs. Addictions are much easier to prevent than to cure, and one questions the wisdom of Professor Burn's apparent acquiescence in heavy smoking until the age of 45 so long as consumption is reduced after that age. For a heavy smoker this is a near impossibility; it is far better never to have begun. But, already, many responsible people do not offer the young cigarettes as well as food and drink. Governments are in a quandary, for most derive much revenue from tobacco. The British people pay about £1,000 million a year in taxes on tobacco, and if anti-smoking campaigns were successful some source of revenue to replace this would have to be found. Nevertheless restrictions on smoking in theatres and public transport have been encouraged, and money has been provided through local authorities for anti-smoking clinics and for anti-smoking posters; restrictions on cigarette advertising on television were imposed in August, 1965. In the United States since 1966 all cigarette cartons must carry a warning of risk to health.

If those who make public policy could harness the formidable forces of persuasion to convince the young that smoking is no part of the grown-up image, the masculine image, but belongs to the middle-aged world of round bellies and bald pates the battle would be half won and by the turn of the century deaths from lung cancer could have returned to a base-line.

There is some evidence that this may be beginning, that the tide may be starting to turn. In his annual report for 1965 the Chief Medical Officer of the Ministry of Health[1] claimed that fewer adolescents were smoking and that in general in 1964 a million fewer people were smoking than would have been expected from extrapolation of the figures for 1961. However, two years later he had returned to his earlier pessimism.

Smoking, heavy cigarette smoking, though the predominant cause of lung cancer, is not the only cause. It occurs in non-smokers and it occurs more often in town-dwellers than in countrymen. Some factor in atmospheric pollution has been suspected of being a carcinogen, or perhaps a co-carcinogen, but as yet this is uncertain.

Dental Caries

There is the clearest evidence that sugar which remains in the mouth long enough to begin being broken down is the main cause of dental decay. The teeth of British children improved during the war when sweets were scarce but have deteriorated since. Over one-third of 13 year-olds have teeth damaged by caries.[2] Sweet-eating is the obvious cause and that this can happen to adults, too, is illustrated in a letter to *The Lancet*.[3] As an aid to giving up smoking a man of twenty resorted to sucking mint sweets. Within 18 months his teeth, previously healthy, developed more than fifty carious lesions.

For once, "stress" has not been implicated, but the illness does have a social aspect. It has been plainly shown that fluorides in the diet can help to prevent caries. The fluoridation of water supplies, a sensible public health measure and strongly supported by the

[1] *Annual Report of the Chief Medical Officer of the Ministry of Health.* (H.M.S.O. London, 1966).
[2] *Brit. Med. J.*, (1965). **ii**, 1197.
[3] Berwick, W. A. (1965). *Lancet*, **ii**, 955.

Ministry of Health, is the only practical way, apart from discouraging sweet-eating, of preventing British children from having six million teeth filled and another million extracted every year. Yet it has been and continues to be opposed by a few zealots for personal liberty in a campaign which only England could provide.

Addiction

This is a peculiarly baffling subject. Every society, it seems, has its accepted drugs of addiction—tea, coffee, tobacco, alcohol in Western

TABLE 7

Drug	Craving	Abstinence Syndrome	Tolerance	Toxic Effects	Placebo Effect	Remarks
Caffeine (tea, coffee)	+	O	O	O	+	
Tobacco	++	O	+	++	+	Lung cancer and other cancers, Bronchitis, Coronary disease.
Alcohol	++	+	++	+++	O	Serious effects on physical and mental health in the long run.
Morphine, Heroin, etc.	+++	+++	+++	O	O	Little toxicity but self injection very liable to lead to infection, abscesses, hepatitis—often fatal.
Barbiturates	++	+	++	+	+	
Amphetamines	++	O	+++	++	++	Psychosis not uncommon
Non-barbiturate hypnotics	+	+	++	+	+	
Cocaine	++	O	+	+	O	
Marijuana	++	O	O	O	O	
Lysergic acid diethylamide (LSD)	+ or O	O	+	++	?	Precipitation of psychosis or suicide. Possible genetic damage.

societies and other drugs elsewhere, marijuana,[1] peyotl, opium or cocaine. They have a variety of effects, stimulant, hallucinogenic, favouring contemplation, euphorising, or increasing extraversion as

[1] Marijuana (hashish, Indian hemp, cannabis indica, reefers, pot, rope, weed, gear, grass, etc.).

the case may be; in moderation they are valued and approved by society. But many of them are liable to abuse either by unstable individuals or, when society itself is under strain, by many more.

Each drug seems fairly harmless in its natural cultural habitat but can have devastating effects in inappropriate groups. Marijuana, used without harm by jazz musicians in the United States, can be misused by teenagers in a cellar in London; and regular heavy drinking in London's clubland is not the same thing as traders introducing alcohol to tribesmen in West Africa. Or, was the alcohol so devastating because the tribesmen were already detribalised; and does this mean that those teenagers are desocialised? Or perhaps modern experimentation with drugs in youth is, as described in the previous chapter, an exploration of a new frontier, a latter-day equivalent of youthful rock climbing and pot-holing—and just as dangerous.

In Britain in 1915 newly affluent munition workers, by their excessive drinking, quickly forced society to extend the Defence of the Realm Act so that the state could control the sale and supply of alcohol in the neighbourhood of these factories. Somewhat the same situation, with abuse of heroin, the amphetamines, and the hallucinogens, is forcing legislative action in the 1960s.[1] Nevertheless, though the growth of drug abuse, its infectiousness and its epidemic quality, is specifically of our time, its social significance is utterly obscure. Sociological theory can produce no firm answers. *Tot homines quot sententiae.*

Doctors have long been accustomed to treating the toxic effects of alcohol and other addictive drugs and to lessening the painful effects of abstinence. They are now expected by society, increasingly inclined to regard addiction in itself as a disease, to try to treat the addiction. Nor is this all. Mid-century medicine must contend with the effects of the pharmaceutical revolution, for many of the industry's discoveries, the barbiturates, the amphetamines, the synthetic pain killing drugs, have turned out to be powerfully addictive.

In 1964 the World Health Organisation's Expert Committee on Addiction-producing Drugs[2] favoured the conception of "drug-dependence" to replace the opprobrious terms addiction and habituation. This state of dependence can arise, the committee says, from the use of a drug either continuously or periodically. It has

---

[1] At the same time pressure was building up for the relaxation of the law relating to marijuana. Because this substance has no known medical uses or medical consequences, it is not discussed further in this book.

[2] WHO. *Tech. Rep.*, no. 273. (Geneva, 1964).

three aspects: psychological dependence or craving; physical dependence or the state in which withdrawal of the drug produces a crop
of bodily symptoms, different for each drug—an abstinence syndrome; and tolerance, the need for the dose to be increased in order
to produce the desired effect. In addition, many of these drugs are
toxic in the high doses used by those who are dependent. Some, too,
can never have their effects mimicked by dummy tablets—the
placebo effect; others can.

In Table 7 a number of drugs on which large numbers of people
are dependent have been assessed separately in these five respects.
But in each respect it is not only the quality of the drug that is
important—in some the physiological and psychological qualities
of the person who becomes dependent matter as much or even more.
The drug itself is of paramount importance in causing both the
abstinence syndrome and toxic effects. It is said that three weeks of
regular heroin injections would render anybody physically dependent
on the drug. Tolerance is an ill-understood subject and differences
between individuals in the ease with which it grows are not confined
to this group of drugs. Clearly both the drug and the person matter,
as they do indeed in deciding whether a drug-dependent person
responds to dummy tablets. No placebo can be substituted for
morphine, but in one group of amphetamine-addicts 43% reported
an enhanced mood after having dummy tablets.[1]

It is the psychological dependence, however, which is most
influenced by personal factors. All these drugs can do one or more
of the following: diminish anxiety; relieve depression and induce
euphoria; stimulate; disinhibit; remove fatigue; abolish pain;
produce the "sent" experience. Those who become dependent on
them have one or more of these handicaps—chronic tension, chronic
unhappiness, chronic pain, chronic shyness, or inferiority feelings—
and they seek relief. But to say this is only to scratch the surface of
the problem, the roots of which lie deep in society.

This century has seen the introduction of a host of new synthetic
drugs on which people can become dependent. Some of these are
pain-relieving drugs, such as pethidine, methadone and dextromora-
mide, which give rise to a morphine-type of dependence with a
severe abstinence syndrome. Others, the barbiturates, amphetamine,
the non-barbiturate sedatives and hypnotics and even aspirin and
the cortisone group of drugs, produce different types of dependence.
Almost invariably a claim is made when the drug is introduced that
it is non-addictive, but soon this claim proves false. The ampheta-

[1] Wilson, C. W. M. and Beacon, S. (1964), *Brit. J. Addiction*, **60**, 81.

mines,[1] first introduced in 1935 and found to be useful in the treatment of a variety of conditions ranging from obesity to bedwetting, were regarded as harmless for twenty years or more. Since then, and particularly in the last five years, it has become plain that this group of drugs not uncommonly produce a psychosis resembling schizophrenia. Moreover, those dependent on it can develop a tolerance to a dose of more than one hundred times the ordinary therapeutic dose. There is no doubt that abuse of the drug is widespread, and as a result of one investigation[2] in Newcastle upon Tyne in 1960 it was estimated that at least two people in every thousand were dependent on this drug or on an amphetamine-barbiturate mixture such as Drinamyl ("purple hearts"). These were mainly married women in the age-group 36–45. The medical indications for the drug are in fact few, far fewer than could account for the 100 million amphetamine tablets prescribed by doctors in Britain in 1965. The newer antidepressant drugs used in psychiatry—the imipramine and monoamine-oxidase inhibitor groups—seem so far to be free of "dependence" risks, though patients may become dependent on them in the same sense as a diabetic is dependent on insulin. They can bring a patient's mood back to normal, but they cannot enhance the mood of a normal person—the secret of amphetamine's charm.

This drug is prominent, too, in that alarming new development in Britain—teenage drug dependence.[3] The ink of the Brain[4] Committee's report in 1961 was hardly dry before its reassuring conclusions were challenged by an epidemic of teenage drug-taking. The committee at that time felt justified in saying (of amphetamine): "we have formed the impression that, while serious cases of addiction arise from time to time, such abuse is not widespread." The alarm was sounded by laymen, for psychiatrists see only the rare case who becomes psychotic, and the teenager who takes "purple hearts" or smokes reefers only at weekends does not regard himself as ill and shuns doctors and clinics.[5] The drugs known by colourful names— "black bombers", "sweeties", "dixies", "red and green bombers", and "French blues"—are seldom obtained on medical prescriptions, unless they are forged. No one has any accurate knowledge of the number of teenagers who abuse amphetamine. The author of an

[1] Amphetamine (Benzedrine), dextro-amphetamine (Dexedrine), methyl-amphetamine (Methedrine), phenmetrazine (Preludin). There are more than 40 preparations on the market in Britain that contain amphetamine. *Prescribers' Journal.* ed. Hunt, J. L. (H.M.S.O. London, 1965), vol. 4. no. 6.
[2] Kiloh, L. G. and Brandon, S. (1962), *Brit. Med. J.*, **ii**, 40.
[3] Scott, P. D. and Willcox, D. R. C. (1965), *Brit. J. Psychiat.*, **111**, 865.
[4] The Interdepartmental Committee on Drug Addiction.
[5] Connell, P. H. (1965), *Proc. Roy. Soc. Med.*, **58**, 409.

article in *The Times* in December, 1965[1] estimated that in and around London a figure of 10,000 is credible as a minimum. Now that the habit has spread beyond inner London to the outer suburbs and to other cities a national figure of several times this is plausible.

To what extent is this misuse harmful and dangerous? At least these teenagers are largely uninterested in alcohol, and sexual promiscuity is not associated with this kind of social drug-taking. Apart from the small risk of psychosis and of violent crime committed in response to persecutory ideas most authors see the main danger to lie in the graduation of a few experimenters with these "soft" drugs to "hard" ones of the morphine type, notably heroin, either alone or combined with cocaine or methylamphetamine.

There is some evidence that this has happened.[2] Until 1959 the number of known addicts to morphine-type drugs in Britain was small and stationary. It was reasonable to suppose that there were very few addicts not "known" to the Home Office; most addicts were middle-aged and had either acquired their addiction in the course of treatment, or were members of professions with easy access to these drugs. The total number was of the order of 450, of whom 68 were dependent on heroin.

By 1966 the number of known addicts to these "hard" drugs had risen to 1,349. Of these 899 were addicted to heroin—a thirteen-fold increase in seven years. Moreover, of the 179 new addicts to heroin in 1965, 77 were obtaining supplies without going to doctors. In 1966 as compared with 1964 there was an increase in those under the age of twenty from 40 to 329 and of these all but 12 were dependent on heroin. In 1959, in contrast, only three were teenagers. These changes and the further increase in 1967 are illustrated in Chart VII.

The scale of the problem in Britain is still minute compared with

---

[1] *The Times*, 20 December, 1965.
[2] In this section I have relied on a number of sources which include:
Bewley, T. (1965), *Lancet*, **i**, 808.
Bewley, T. (1965), *Brit. Med. J.*, **ii**, 1284.
Bewley, T. (1966), *Bull. Narcot.*, **18**, 4. 1.
Bewley, T. et al. (1968), *Brit. Med. J.* **i**, 725.
Chein, I., Gerard, D. L., Lee, R. S. and Rosenfeld, E. *Narcotics, Delinquency and Social Policy—The Road to H.* (Tavistock Publications, 1964).
Clark, J. A. (1965), *Proc. Roy. Soc. Med.*, **58**, 412.
Edwards, G., (1967), *Brit. Med. J.*, **iii**, 425.
Hansard, 30 June, 1966.
Glatt, M. M. (1965), *Lancet*, **ii**, 171.
Glatt, M. M., Pittman, D. J., Gillespie, D. G., and Hills, D. R. *The Drug Scene in Great Britain.* (Edward Arnold. London, 1967).
James, I. P. (1967), *Brit. J. Addict.*, **62**.
Kolb, L. *Drug Addiction.* (Springfield, Illinois, 1962).
Lancet, 21 March, 1964, p. 649.
Schur, E. M. *Narcotic Addiction in Britain and America.* (Tavistock Publications. London, 1963).

the United States, where even cautious estimates of the number of addicts to hard drugs range between 50,000 and 100,000; the latest British figures faintly suggest that the epidemic rise is starting to flatten out and that in scale the problem will not resemble America's.

The increase in drug addiction

Chart VII

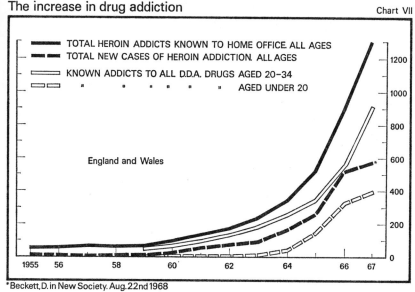

TOTAL HEROIN ADDICTS KNOWN TO HOME OFFICE. ALL AGES
TOTAL NEW CASES OF HEROIN ADDICTION. ALL AGES
KNOWN ADDICTS TO ALL D.D.A. DRUGS AGED 20–34
"   "   "   "   "   " AGED UNDER 20

England and Wales

1955 56 58 60 62 64 66 67

*Beckett, D. in New Society. Aug. 22nd 1968
Source: Reports to the United Nations on the working of the International Treaties on Narcotic Drugs 1954–67. Bewley, T. (1966) Bull. Narcot. 18. 4. 1.

As with alcohol, the treatment of dependence of the morphine-heroin type divides itself into two phases. The withdrawal phase lasting a few weeks is simple. "Cold Turkey", the abrupt cutting off of supplies, is cruel and unnecessary and is only too likely to discourage a relapsed patient from ever undergoing it again. Withdrawal must be gradual and it is likely to be achieved best in hospital, though one American expert claims some success with out-patient treatment. Here lies the difficulty. At present, again as with alcohol, no powers of compulsory admission exist unless the patient has become psychotic. Inevitably, because neither alcoholics nor addicts early on think of themselves as ill, before a first effort at treatment is attempted the alcoholic's addiction has often been established for years and he has drunk his money and his job away and his family into despair. So, too, with the heroin-dependent the addiction is well-established. If he belongs to the stabilised group, able to obtain a regular supply from a doctor, he is lucky, but he is continually under suspicion and under pressure to reduce demand. If not, if he belongs to the new group of younger addicts dependent on illicit sources, he is inevitably condemned to move in a semi-criminal subculture whose *mores* he must accept. This makes his eventual cure the more difficult and unlikely.

The second phase of treatment, after withdrawal is complete, is both difficult and unsuccessful. Psychological probing to uncover the causes of the individual's dependence, individual and group psychotherapy, aversion therapy, rehabilitation, follow-up—these are the methods in use at present. Even for those whose addiction arose in the course of treatment and for "professional" addicts the recovery rates reported from various countries seldom reach 30%; for nontherapeutic addicts the United States figures, unreliable as they are in this field, suggest that fewer than 10% do not relapse, and such figures as are available concerning this new problem in Britain are certainly little better.[1]

Until very recently the British policy of keeping the management of addiction firmly in medical hands was the envy of American reformers. Ever since the United States Harrison Act of 1914, the unintended consequence of which was to make it impossible for doctors to treat addicts unless they were prepared to have their good faith questioned in court, the Americans have handled the addiction problem largely as a penal matter. In a sense they can claim a little success. In 1914 there were estimated to be about 200,000 addicts in the United States, perhaps more; opiates could be obtained cheaply without prescription, and many patent medicines contained large amounts. Today there are fewer addicts, certainly; but this reduction has been achieved at the cost of creating by legislation a new army of criminals. Ironically, two fairly recent American books praising the British system were published in 1962 at a time when the deficiencies of this system of medical control were just beginning to be apparent. The "professional" and "therapeutic" middle-aged addict, who had reasonably free access to supplies to satisfy his own need, was very seldom a focus from which addiction spread.

The weakness of the British system was that a few doctors, either from greed or from misguided sympathy, over-prescribed for the younger addict. He[2] had progressed to opiates often from other drugs and practised his addiction in café and club society rather than alone. He obtained supplies from friends, who asked for and got far

---

[1] Advocates of replacement therapy with methadone, itself a dependence-producing drug, claim much better results in selected addicts. (Dole, V. P., Nyswander, M. E. and Kreek, M. J. 1965, *J. Amer. Med. Ass.*, **193**, 646 and 1966, *Arch. Intern. Med.*, **118**, 304).

[2] There are about three boys for every girl.

more heroin on prescriptions from doctors than they needed for themselves and who could live without working on the proceeds of selling the excess. Later he might find a doctor willing to supply him, exaggerated his need, and himself made a profit from encouraging some acquaintance to start "mainlining". "Epidemic" is hardly too strong a word to describe the effects of this abuse in the last few years.

If the American error is to be avoided in Britain, it is clearly essential to keep the treatment of addicts in medical hands however unsatisfactory and unreliable they prove to be as patients and however disappointing their response to treatment may seem. Britain's new legislation and the regulations accompanying it give rise to some misgiving. The aim is to confine the prescription of heroin to doctors working in newly set up treatment centres and in mental hospitals, to try to ensure that the addict has only just enough heroin for his own needs, to prevent impersonation, and to offer again and again longer term treatment in mental hospitals rather than in treatment centres to rehabilitate patients from whom the drug has been withdrawn.

We are delicately poised. If such a system is run too loosely, too kindly, too tolerantly, we shall be back where we started with addicts, and pseudo-addicts, having sufficient heroin to sell to create new addicts. More probably the system will fail or partially fail from proving too rigid to contain the problem completely. Mental hospitals may find addicts too disruptive to their ordinary work; addicts themselves may become intolerant of the rules and the rigidity—for they can be very difficult people; or doctors may become impatient and discouraged by the frequency of relapse. If this happens, and if an increasing proportion of the addicted are forced outside the medical system, black market prices could rise (from the present £1 per grain), non-addicted peddlers appear and violent crime could increase. Until now in Britain, because heroin has been cheap, addicts unattached to any doctor have had little difficulty in obtaining it. A failure of the new system might lead straight on to a repetition of the American experience.

There is controversy about whether compulsory treatment is justified or not. Certainly, compulsory admission is not possible under the present mental treatment laws unless words are made to bear meanings that they were never intended to have. There is a case, however, for regarding compulsory admission as justifiable once or twice in an effort to cure. If this fails nothing remains but to try to stabilise the patient, perhaps on methadone (which has the advantage of being active by mouth in twice daily doses), in the hope that, as with so much disturbed behaviour due to personality disorder, the addiction might subside when the patient reaches his thirties—if he survives.[1]

As a postscript it is worth remarking that the familiar combination of heroin with cocaine has given place to combination now with intravenous methylamphetamine (Methedrine), not only in Britain but in Sweden also. Supply of this drug in intravenous form has therefore been restricted to hospitals.

This seems to be an appropriate place to mention lysergic acid diethylamide and the other hallucinogenic[2] drugs. Like the amphetamines, heroin and marijuana, these drugs have been misused and in the same sort of circumstances and for the same reasons first in the United States and more recently in Britain and elsewhere.

Naturally occurring hallucinogens have been used in religious practices for centuries; the peyote cactus (mescaline), the teonanacatl mushroom (psilocybin) and the ololiuqui or morning glory (d-lysergic acid) all originate in Mexico. Since the beginning of this century, too, these natural products and their active principles have been used in psychiatric research. They produce extraordinary disturbances of perception vividly described by Aldous Huxley[3]—disordered sense of time, visual hallucinations, and experiences which some find to be mystical, even transcendental. As many find the experience extremely unpleasant. Hallucinogens, particularly since Dr Hofmann produced lysergic acid diethylamide in 1938 and accidentally discovered its well-nigh incredible potency in 1943, have found a use in medicine. Some psychiatrists are impressed by this drug as an adjunct to psychotherapy as it seems capable of making repressed material rapidly available; others are wary of its capacity to produce psychotic symptoms and behaviour that may not be so readily reversed by the passage of time or by phenothiazine drugs as they should be in theory. In fact there is a slowly accumulating dossier of disasters—the precipitation of psychosis with paranoid symptoms in the unstable, the recurrence of psychotic symptoms days afterwards when the patient may well not be under medical observation, suicide, and at least one murder. According to Dr Cohen,[4] who in 1960 sent a questionnaire to sixty-two European and North American investigators with experience of using mescaline or LSD on 5,000 people, the incidence of prolonged psychosis is about 2 per 1,000 patients; and

---

[1] 13% mortality in the first year after discharge from hospital is reported in one study. (Bewley, T. 1968, *Brit. Med. J.*, **i,** 727).

[2] Also called psychotomimetic or psychedelic drugs.

[3] Huxley, A. *The Doors of Perception.* (Chatto and Windus. London, 1954).

[4] Cohen, S. *Drugs of Hallucination.* (Secker and Warburg. London, 1964).

of suicide and attempted suicide 1·6 per 1,000. But since these drugs have been used for kicks in unstable or sick people without medical supervision the incidence in them is almost certainly much higher.

Lately there have been reports that LSD can produce genetic damage, but this possibility is still unconfirmed.

Hallucinogens are obviously potentially dangerous and every effort should be made to restrict their use to research into schizophrenia and therapy of the neuroses. Even in treating patients doctors will have to be extremely cautious not to transgress the rule of *primum non nocere*.

Attempted Suicide

For a variety of reasons official statistics on the number of suicides and on suicide rates are unreliable. They tend to underestimate the true figures, but to differing degrees in different countries. The methods of collecting the figures vary and, in at least some Roman Catholic and Moslem countries, every effort is made to arrive at some other verdict to spare the family's feelings. Trends within one country, however, have more validity, particularly if account is taken of any change in the age-composition of the population, for the likelihood of suicide increases with age. In England and Wales suicide rates for males since the war have remained more or less stationary (at 13–15 per 100,000) and are well below the high rates recorded in the nineteen thirties; for women the rates (at about 9 per 100,000), while still below those for men, are rising, a characteristic of the figures for many Western countries.[1]

Reliable figures for suicidal attempts not resulting in death are even more difficult to obtain. Professor Stengel[2] has estimated on the basis of his own and other work that in Britain and the United States the number of attempts is six to eight times that of achieved suicides, at least in towns. His most recent survey in Sheffield[3] showed a ratio of 9·7 to 1 in 1960–61. This estimate of perhaps 40,000 in Britain and 130,000 in the United States takes no account of the sizeable but unknown number of attempts that occur without subsequent admission to hospital or a call for medical help.

No comparison can be made with earlier years—the figures are impossible to estimate—but it is common knowledge among doctors

---

[1] In 1965 in England and Wales the number of male suicides fell below 3,000 for the first time in thirteen years and the rate for males and females at 10·8 per 100,000 was the lowest since 1953. In 1967 the improved trend continued (male 11·6; female 8·0).
[2] Stengel, E. *Suicide and Attempted Suicide.* (Penguin Books. London, 1964).
[3] Parkin, D. and Stengel, E. (1965), *Brit. Med. J.* ii, 133.

that this is largely a new and postwar phenomenon. Indeed figures from Edinburgh[1] suggest tentatively that admissions from this cause are now five times what they were in the late 1940s. Patients admitted to hospital after attempting suicide make heavy demands on medical and nursing time and skill, not only because a proportion of the more serious cases require sophisticated techniques of resuscitation but also because of the need, after recovery, for painstaking psychiatric and social enquiry and help. This special group of people who have made one or more suicidal attempts contains twice as many women as men, particularly women below the age of 45; throughout the country there may at any time be as many as half-a-million of them—in the United States there may well be 2 million;[2] they present all kinds of marital and domestic, social and alcoholic problems and a proportion will injure themselves again. Perhaps 10% will ultimately commit suicide.

Criticism has lately been made of the term "attempted suicide" by Professor Kessel[3] on the grounds of inaccuracy. Of his group of 522 patients in Edinburgh only 20% could be said to have "done all they could to encompass their deaths". The remainder had other motives and did not expect death. His alternative term "self-poisoning", however, is rather too restricted. It leaves out of account, among those who make unsuccessful attempts at self-injury, a group of perhaps 5% who adopt other methods than the use of domestic gas and poisons, although their motives may be as mixed. The point is well-taken whatever one calls the phenomenon—attempted suicide, self-poisoning, intentional self-injury. More often than not many of the features of the act are not compatible with self-destruction: warnings are uttered; some tablets are left in the bottle; other people are at hand or expected; there is little money in the gas meter; windows are left open; and occasionally tablets are swallowed actually in the presence of others. What purports to be an act of self-destruction has elements both of aggressive behaviour towards others and of an appeal for help from those who are near and from the wider community.

This is not to suggest that a class of "genuine" attempts is to be sharply distinguished from a class of bogus ones in which deliberate "play-acting" and conscious manipulation of other people take place. On the contrary, as Professor Stengel has written, "Many suicidal attempts and quite a few suicides are carried out in the mood 'I don't

[1] Kessel, N. (1965), *Brit. Med. J.*, **ii**, 1265 and 1336.
[2] Dublin, L. T. *Suicide: a Sociological and Statistical Study.* (Ronald Press Co. New York, 1963).
[3] Kessel, N., loc. cit.

care whether I live or die';" and again, "Uncertainty of outcome
i.e. from the point of view of the person committing the act, is a
common feature of most attempts at suicide". The very uncertainty
seems to be a crucial element in many. The act is a gamble, an
ordeal, a test of one's standing with the gods. This aspect of suicidal
attempts and the dicing-with-death element in human psychology
have been discussed by Professor Cohen[1] in his studies of behaviour
in conditions of uncertainty.

In his report on self-poisoning in Edinburgh Professor Kessel shows
that the use of non-drug poisons—disinfectants and corrosives—had
steadily diminished since the war; aspirin, which now accounts for
12% of the admissions, is slowly increasing and is used mainly by the
young; barbiturates are much the commonest drugs employed
(55%); and other drugs—mainly tranquillisers, non-barbiturate
sedatives and anti-depressants—are increasingly used and now
account for a quarter of the admissions. If it is true that an "ordeal"
element reinforces the "appeal" factor in many suicidal attempts,
aspirin, barbiturates and these newer drugs are ideal for the purpose.
Older methods of self-destruction, the use of corrosive poisons,
throwing oneself out of a window or in front of a train, hanging,
drowning, cutting blood vessels were a great deal too certain of
success to be used if the aim is to commit one's life to chance. With
these newer methods there is no pain, though the sheer physical discomfort of swallowing a hundred tablets must be considerable; there
is time for loved ones (or hated ones for that matter) to arrive and
for the instruments of society's concern, the police and the doctors,
to be summoned, backed, if need be, by the formidable armoury of
modern medicine. For a small proportion the hovering between life
and death, tended by doctors and nurses and machines, is evidence
that society wants them not to die.

Most doctors resent the time and trouble spent on what to them
seems a wilfully procured diversion of their energy from more important tasks. But is the time spent on resections of lung cancers, on
some of the orthopaedic surgery for road casualties, on dealing with
the ravages of alcohol, and even on the treatment and care of some
middle-aged patients with coronary attacks, better spent, more
deserved, any less wilfully procured?

In no longer regarding attempted suicide as an offence in Britain
since 1961 society has only conformed to what had become the
common view. This is not to say that it now approves of this be-

---

[1] Cohen, J. *Behaviour in Uncertainty*. (Allen and Unwin. London, 1964).

haviour. On the contrary no society could approve of an act whose apparent meaning is so critical of it. The change has come about because the generality of people see other causes behind the façade of the act: mental illness, which can be treated; isolation and other social difficulties, which may be helped; physical ill-health and alcoholic excess which may be more refractory; or a crisis in personal relationships, which the act may help to solve. Obviously, once it has happened doctors, if they can, must resuscitate the patient and, seeing the act as a danger signal, must direct him to where help, medical, psychiatric or social, can be obtained. This happens already in almost every case. But what can be done to prevent such acts?

Authorities differ on what proportion of people who make self-destructive acts give any warning. Professor Stengel says that "the large majority" do so; Professor Kessel found that only a third had done so. Often enough these warnings are ignored, discounted, regarded as empty threats. A large number of attempts are, however, impulsive and made on the spur of the moment. Some of these could probably be prevented if some restriction were placed on the sale of aspirin and if doctors were less lavish in prescribing larger numbers of tablets, particularly barbiturates, at a time. It would be beneficial, too, if people habitually disposed of unused supplies of pills instead of tucking them away in a medicine chest.

An event with such complex causes is not likely to yield to simple remedies. The medical practicioner is already there for those who issue clear warnings, and he is backed by psychiatric clinics and a local mental welfare service. For the religious there is the priest. For others there are the probation officer and a host of voluntary organisations ranging from Marriage Guidance counsellors to the Family Welfare Association. But the increase in self-injury makes it plain that these people and organisations, who often enough help after the act, are not approached before it. If they are not approached, is it because they are often unapproachable? The growth of organisations in various countries to which access is instant, by telephone, is an attempt to reach despairing people who are tempted to suicide. In Britain the Samaritans are trying to fill this role. Their work has been described elsewhere.[1]

Apart from the sensible restriction of ready access to potentially lethal tablets, which incidently might reduce accidental poisoning in children, these modes of social help are all designed to answer the "appeal" implicit in the act of self-injury. Perhaps we shall not get much farther until means are found to deal with the "aggressive"

[1] Stengel, E., op. cit.

component and the "ordeal" aspect. These may well prove far more difficult.

Accidents

In Britain accidents are now the commonest cause of death below the age of 40—accidents in the home, on the road, in industry, in sport, in the air and elsewhere (see Table 8). They burden the hospital services to the extent of 300,000 admissions a year. Altogether there are 24,000 deaths from accidents each year and the figures, particularly for road deaths, have crept upwards. But there is nothing very new about this, and in fact it is only recently, in 1960, that the number of deaths in traffic accidents exceeded the figures of twenty-five years earlier. There is certainly little enough reason to use the words "modern plague" or "epidemic" to imply unusual prevalence. Accidents have been endemic for a very long time, and accidents in the home kill more people, particularly children and old people, than accidents on the road.

TABLE 8

Common causes of death in the first half of life.
Deaths in 1965 (England and Wales) and rank order.

Causes	Age 1–4		Age 5–14		Age 15–24		Age 25–34	
Accident: Motor vehicle	237 }	I	498 }	I	1908 }	I	738 }	I
Others	416 }		393 }		588 }		423 }	
Cancer	332	3	516	2	633	2	1109	2
Infectious diseases	171	5	75		79		103	
Pneumonia	421	2	133	4	118		128	
Vascular lesions of brain. e.g. aneurysm	12		38		90		210	5
Nephritis	11		47		128		123	
Coronary artery disease	2		1		23		244	4
Asthma	37		84	5	152	4	167	
Rheumatic heart disease	2		4		50		169	
Congenital malformation	326	4	247	3	141	5	87	
Suicide	0		3		310	3	520	3
Total	1,967		2,039		4,220		4,021	
Total deaths in each age group.	2,665		2,556		5,007		5,216	

Source: Registrar General's Statistical Review 1965.
Part I. Tables, medical. Table 17.

No doubt because other causes of death have become so much less common in the young, deaths from accidents stand out more prominently. Just how prominently can be seen in Table 8. Medicine and society are paying them more attention and are looking beyond the accident and its consequences to its prior causes. Most accidents are avoidable and their prevention is a fairly new field for preventive medicine, aided by designers and technicians of all kinds. In the home, for example, there is a degree of predictability about accidents that result from unguarded fires, inflammable clothing, attractive tablets left about, boiling saucepans within reach of small children, slippery and uneven floors, and baths that are difficult for the elderly to get into and out of. On the road doctors have taken a hand in pointing out, from their experience of the types of injury sustained, the weak points of vehicle design which, if remedied, would save life and limit human damage. Professor Gissane[1] [2] [3] and his colleagues, for example, in Britain have criticised the flimsy construction, rigid steering wheels and columns, internal projections, weak door latches and absence of seat belts on many modern cars. They say that rear overhang and loads that can shift are dangerous features of lorries, and they plead for both minimum and maximum speeds on motorways as an attempt to reduce the velocity of impact.

In the United States the authorities have insisted on manufacturers complying with stringent new safety standards in car design and with measures to reduce air pollution.

But the improvement to vehicles, to roads and to lighting will achieve little unless there is also an improvement in the prudence and skill of those who use the roads. There is mounting evidence that alcohol is the greatest single cause of death. In Britain 20–30% of drivers involved in fatal accidents had a blood alcohol level of 50 mg per 100 millilitres of blood (by general agreement the upper limit of relative safety). At Christmas the proportion is higher. Nor is the driver solely at fault. Pedestrians who are killed have often been drinking—20% in an investigation in Oslo[4] in 1952–61, 43% in New York City.[5] It seems probable that alcohol plays some part in causing between one-third and one-half of all road deaths. Yet despite a wealth of evidence the changes in legislation and in society's attitude to discourage the drinking driver come very, very slowly.

[1] Gissane, W. (1963), *Lancet*, **ii**, 695.
[2] Gissane, W. and Bull, J. (1961), *Brit. Med. J.*, **i**, 1716.
[3] Gissane, W. and Bull, J. (1964), *Brit. Med. J.*, **i**, 75.
[4] Solheim, K. (1964), *Brit. Med. J.*, **i**, 81.
[5] McCarroll, J. R., Braunstein, P. W., Cooper, W., Helpern, M., Seremetis, M., Wade, P. A. and Weinberg, S. B. (1962), *J.A.M.A.*, **180**, 127.

It is still commonly regarded as "unfair" for the police to lurk outside public houses at closing time.

In October 1967, Britain's Road Safety Act came into force. This makes it an offence to drive with a blood alcohol level of 80 mg per 100 ml or a urine alcohol level of 107 mg per 100 ml. Britain thus comes into line with a number of other countries who have introduced restrictions of this sort. Preliminary results have been encouraging for, as compared with a year before, road deaths since the Act have been reduced by nearly 15%. It looks as though this Act may save over 1,000 deaths a year.

Nevertheless, since the end of the war, deaths from road accidents are creeping up in most countries as are the rates for a unit of population. Chart VIII (pp. 226–7) compares the trend of these rates in ten selected countries with results that may cause surprise.[1]

France, Italy and West Germany have shown a pattern of steeply rising rates as they recovered from the destruction of wartime; in England and Wales the increase has been more modest; in the United States the rate has been held steady. But it is a sobering thought that in these ten countries, with between them a population of 530 millions, in the ten years 1954–1963 938,000 people were killed on the roads—twice as many people as live in Edinburgh.

If Britain is doing fairly well in comparison with some other countries any complacency is entirely out of place, for the total figures of road deaths in England and Wales conceal an epidemic that other countries do not seem to have. There is a large increase in the last ten years in deaths of teenage motor bicyclists and their passengers. For males aged 15–19 the number killed increased almost five-fold between 1953 and 1964. The full facts are shown in Chart IX. From these figures, and from a survey made in 1958 of the ages and mileage of these teenagers,[2] it has been calculated[3] that for every year that a boy owns a motorcycle he has a 2% chance of being killed or seriously injured. This grim fact has wiped out the improvement in mortality from disease achieved in the same age group in the nineteen-fifties.

In spite of various changes—the near universal wearing of crash helmets, the restriction of the use of large machines to those who have passed a driving test—the epidemic continues. A general impression that injuries caused in this way are getting less common and that

[1] These international comparisons are not entirely fair. Countries differ in the definitions they use—death at the site of the accident, death within a week, death within a month. But for any one country the trend is much more meaningful.
[2] Scott, C. and Jackson, S. *Accidents to Young Motor Cyclists*. (London, 1960).
[3] Lee, J. A. H. (1963), *Proc. Roy. Soc. Med.*, **56**, 365.

P

Death rates from motor-vehicle accidents:

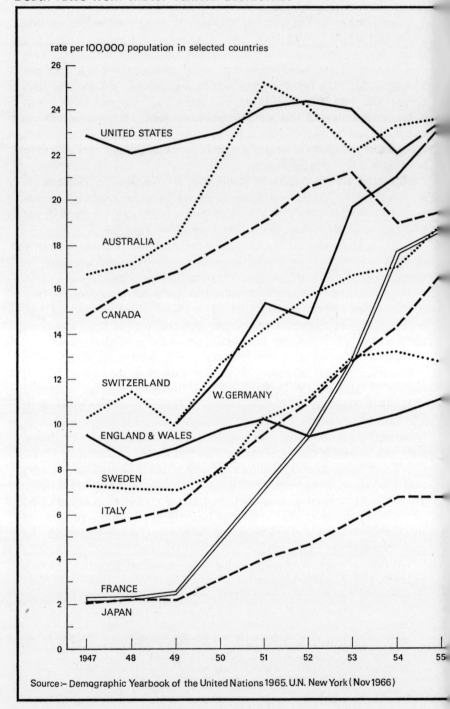

rate per 100,000 population in selected countries

UNITED STATES
AUSTRALIA
CANADA
SWITZERLAND
W. GERMANY
ENGLAND & WALES
SWEDEN
ITALY
FRANCE
JAPAN

1947 48 49 50 51 52 53 54 55

Source:– Demographic Yearbook of the United Nations 1965. U.N. New York (Nov 1966)

Chart VIII

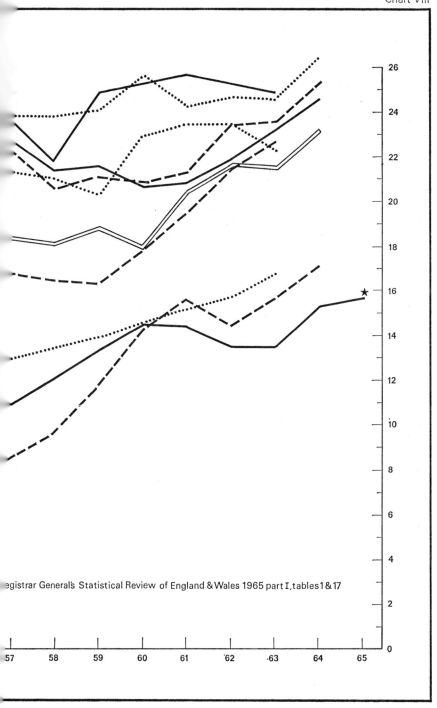

egistrar General's Statistical Review of England & Wales 1965 part I, tables 1 & 17

groups of teenage youths roaming the corridors of hospitals in wheel-
chairs, wearing their leg plasters like battle scars, are less often seen
has yet to be reflected for sure in the deaths recorded in the national

Deaths of motorcyclists and their passengers aged 15–24   Chart IX (a)

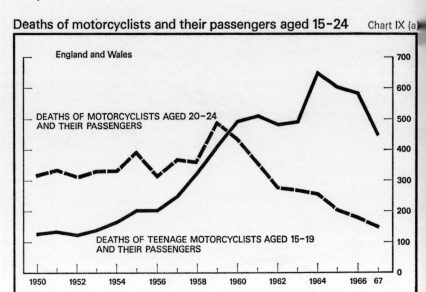

Source: Registrar General's Statistical Reviews. Table 17. I.C.D. E 814, E 815, E 821

Motorcycles (over 60 cc's)   Chart IX (b)

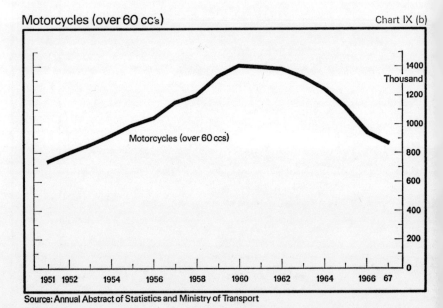

Source: Annual Abstract of Statistics and Ministry of Transport

statistics. Nor is the prospect that with continuing teenage affluence this age-group will gradually shift its allegiance, as have older men, from the motor cycle to the motorcar likely to reduce the number of deaths very much. For, of drivers and riders killed on the roads in 1964, 43% were under 25, and of the total of riders and drivers killed and seriously injured the proportion under 25 years old had risen in three years from 47·9 to 50·7%.

The internal combustion engine helps to increase the mortality of the middle-aged because it discourages exercise. It may also, as has been mentioned, by contributing to atmospheric pollution help to cause lung cancer. For the young it is lethal in other ways. So long as it is confined to its primary purpose of transporting someone from place to place it is comparatively harmless, for the youthful usually get plenty of exercise in any case. It is when a machine is used as an extension of the body image for the expression of status, as a symbol of nascent masculinity, as a weapon in aggressive competition, or as a means of achieving the physiological thrill of acceleration, that it becomes a menace, not only to the rider or driver but also to others who are using the roads for their own, quite different, purposes.

As with arterial disease, addiction and attempted suicide, so with road accident casualties it is the increase affecting the young that is so disturbing. It has been suggested that in teenagers "dicing-with-death" motivation largely underlies both the epidemic of motor-cycle deaths in males and the tablet-swallowing episodes of girls. Medicine can cope, and has always coped, with the results of these injuries, addictions and diseases, but it is becoming plainer that this is not enough and that to try to prevent them is a legitimate part of the new social and preventive medicine. Doctors are needed as well as sociologists, statisticians, psychologists and educationists to track down the causes of the new epidemics, among which violence in its various manifestations, including the battered baby syndrome, may soon be given a place.

CHAPTER ELEVEN

The Need for Change in Medical Education

The previous chapters of this book have uncovered the changed and changing face of medicine in this twentieth century. The chapter headings have proclaimed one by one the major categories of change. In sum the transformation of each feature has been so fundamental, and the relation between them so distorted, as to make the face unrecognisable.

What adaptation has medical education, the training of doctors, made to this transformation of medical practice? How have the curricula of medical students throughout the world been altered to take account of the impact of scientific knowledge, of the defeat of some diseases and the growing importance of others, of exploding populations and ageing populations, and of the basic medical needs of poor countries. The answers are disappointing. Medical education has conspicuously failed to adapt itself to the needs of the varied societies of the mid-twentieth century, and this criticism is as true of the countries of continental Europe, where medical education is more academically based and dominated by universities, as it is of Britain, particularly in London, where medical training is based on an antique apprentice system.[1]

The main defect of the British training has been that as clinical teachers have become more specialised they have tended to create new doctors in their own image, the ideal of the skilled specialist. The defect of the European system is best expressed in the phrase: "it hardly seems logical to entrust the professional education of men who may never practise medicine in an institution exclusively to those who never work outside it."[2]

It is true that there has been a plethora of reports, plans, conferences, recommendations. More than ten years ago an American critic said: "No country has produced so many wise reports on the improvement

[1] Stevens, R. *Medical Practice in Modern England.* (Yale University Press. New Haven and London, 1966).
[2] Miller, H. (1966), *Lancet,* **ii,** 647.

of medical education as Great Britain, and no country has done so little about it." There have since been the General Medical Council's wise recommendations[1] and, wisest of all, the recommendations of the Royal Commission on Medical Education.[2] This met well-nigh every criticism made since the war and incorporates most of the constructive suggestions that have been made as well. But it is still true to say that a medical student can qualify in Britain without having had a single lecture in psychology, that the teaching of preventive medicine has not changed in thirty years, and that there is still only one professor of general practice in all the universities of Britain.

The United States has moved further. In less than a decade more than a dozen new medical schools, each with its own and often unique curriculum, have begun training students. More are on the way. "Core" curricula, varied individual choice, integration of clinical and scientific teaching, opportunities for students to do research, the recognition of postgraduate training as a continuing responsibility of a university—these developments are not plans as they are in Britain, but are happening in various medical schools. Yet, a critic can still say: "In a very general way a standard curriculum has held sway in American schools for more than half a century."[3]

Criticisms of hidebound courses is heard all over the Western world. Elsewhere it is being recognised that Western systems of medical education are not necessarily suited to the needs of developing countries: "it has been too readily assumed that the pattern of Western medical education (an invisible export in imperial days) with its emphasis on the medical school and curative medicine was the correct one for developing countries with their over-riding need for community care and preventive medicine."[4]

Should these countries aim at producing doctors on the Western model at a cost of £6–7,000 each—with the risk that this will be lost if the basically trained doctor departs perhaps permanently for postgraduate training elsewhere? Or would limited resources be better spent in training a larger number of semi-skilled technicians for limited jobs—pest control, birth control, the teaching of hygiene?

The best way in which present deficiencies in medical education can be shown is to ask for answers to a few questions, questions that arise directly from the material of this book. For this purpose it is not necessary to go into great detail or to enter into current controversy

---

[1] *Recommendations as to Basic Medical Education*. General Medical Council. (London, 1967).
[2] *Report of the Royal Commission on Medical Education*. (H.M.S.O. London, 1968).
[3] Jacobson, E. D. (1967), *J. Med. Educ.*, **42,** 1081.
[4] Allen, R. B. (1966), at Third International World Conference on Medical Education. New Delhi, in *Brit. J. Med. Educ.*, **i,** 99.

to more than a limited extent. The answers apply by and large to Britain, but many apply elsewhere too and they are present answers, not the hypothetical and conditional ones that might be true in a few years' time if plans lead to action.

Seven Questions

1. *Has medical education adapted itself to the vast increase in scientific knowledge?*

The answer here must be No. The range of basic sciences relevant to the study of modern medicine has expanded. The new list includes, among others, mathematics, sociology, genetics and psychology; Dr Harlem in Norway, planner of a new medical school, would add ecology and social psychology.[1]

Every doctor needs a grasp of mathematical skill as part of his critical equipment to enable him to understand medical statistics, epidemiology, the results of drug trials, multifactorial inheritance, computers, and the complex causal networks in social medicine and psychiatry. But if new subjects are to be introduced something must go, and it has proved exceptionally difficult to induce those who now have a hold on the student's time to relinquish any part of it. The most obvious places to prune are in the premedical and preclinical phases. Is it really important for a doctor to be able to describe the life-cycle and reproductive system of the Scots pine or to dissect out an ovary of an earthworm? Must he spend five terms dissecting every part of the human body and learn the origin and insertion of every single muscle? Some histology could probably be discarded as well and be left, together with detailed anatomy, to reappear after qualification for the budding surgeon. The danger that such a broadening of the course would encourage superficiality at the expense of depth is smaller than it is in the present courses, where the requirement that the student should commit to memory a huge assembly of facts can obscure for him the general principles of the subject.

Indeed, the more radical suggestion has been made that the premedical years should be spent in studying a wide range of subjects—one or more in honours depth—for a B.Sc. degree in human biology or a tripos in medical sciences. Anatomy, physiology and pharmacology would be joined by social anthropology, psychology, genetics and statistics, and the course might well prove suitable for other students who were not embarking on a medical career. Such a course

[1] Harlem, O. K. (1968), *Brit. Med. J.*, **i,** 441.

might end the isolation of the medical student, who, especially in London, belongs at present much more to a particular medical school than he does to the university. With long hours spent in laboratories and in the dissecting room, and forced to amass a formidable amount of detail in subjects that are hardly of general interest, he is often regarded by his non-medical fellow-students, if he ever meets them, as a frank bore.

2. *Has medical education kept pace with the scientific techniques of clinical medicine and with the drug revolution?*

The answer is certainly Yes. Here we have the romance of modern medicine, its new divining rods and its therapeutic marvels. Moreover because the non-academic clinical chief is actively engaged in clinical practice he is fully up-to-date.

But there is a paradox. To start with the student is rightly taught that the essence of good medicine is to take a thorough history from the patient and then to examine him systematically and comprehensively. He next learns that his chief relies less and less on unaided clinical examination and more and more on extensive laboratory investigation before making a diagnosis and embarking on treatment. Later, in general practice, the new doctor can find himself at a loss, cut off, as he should not be but often is, from access to all but the simplest X-ray and laboratory aids. He has been trained, he finds, too much for hospital medicine, too little for the un-backed-up conditions of general practice.

3. *Has medical education come to terms with specialisation and the centrifugal forces in medicine?*

By no means. Many of the chiefs who teach students in their clinical years have become superspecialists. A surgeon may deal only with chest surgery, a physician only with neurological or endocrinological cases. Even though this danger is well recognised by his teachers, the student's experience may be thereby distorted. He may lack experience of other common conditions.

The chief, too, presumably an enthusiast for his subject, may well find it difficult to limit his teaching to what the basic doctor should know. It is true that much teaching that a student receives is from registrars and others who have access to a wider range of case material. But teaching hospitals attract the unusual case, the complex case, the case requiring super-special techniques of investigation. It is thus questionable whether more than a small part of a student's clinical training ought to take place in a teaching hospital at all.

4. *Has medical education taken account of developments in preventive and social medicine?*

Again the answer must be hardly at all. Students in Britain thirty years ago were given six or eight lectures on public health. Some visits were arranged to a factory or perhaps to a sewage farm. These were optional and poorly attended. Often the student thought that his time could be better used in revising for his examinations. Today the situation incredibly is essentially the same in many places though some schools—Newcastle[1] is one—are exceptions, and doubtless many departments—maternity, for example, and paediatrics—stress the importance of the preventive aspects of their work.

Probably more than half the students will practise after registration in the community rather than in hospital; yet with rare exceptions— Edinburgh possesses the only university department of general practice—little or no teaching of either this or of public health practice goes on in Britain's medical schools. No one explores with the student the changed role of the general practitioner, his relatively diminishing importance as a personal physician, his function as a filter and as a portal of access to expensive and much esteemed technical advances, and what should be his new role in the front-line prevention of disease. The new doctor in general practice finds himself ill-prepared for co-operation with local health and welfare services, or with the school medical service. But such co-operation is essential in maternity and child welfare, and in the care of the mentally subnormal, the mentally ill, the old and chronic sick, and the tuberculous. In hospital the young doctor has been taught to appreciate the "good teaching case", full of physical signs: cavitated tuberculosis of the lung; the extraordinary colour of a patient with severe pernicious anaemia; or new cases presenting with advanced cancer. He will seldom have been taught to regard these as a reproach either to the patient or to medicine—as something that should never have happened. We all pay lip service to prevention and to early diagnosis, and therefore he should welcome the perfection of screening techniques for the presymptomatic diagnosis of a lengthening list of diseases provided they have been established as of value. The student should be taught that as a practitioner later he will be ideally placed both to help by persuasion to keep the population in a state of high immunity to infectious diseases and, by identifying the high-risk case, to play an essential part in the success of screening programmes.

The pat answer to criticisms of the content of the student's curri-

[1] Walker, J. H., and Barnes, H. G. (1966), *Brit. Med. J.*, **ii**, 1129.

culum is to say: "Yes, these things are important and he can learn them later. As an undergraduate he must learn to take a comprehensive history, examine the patient systematically and arrive at a diagnosis." A particular technique can certainly be acquired later; but not necessarily the principle that prevention is better than cure. As with a belief in the virtue of the scientific method this maxim can hardly be emphasised too early. No plan to regard general practice as a specialty in its own right and needing specific postgraduate training[1] can compensate for neglect to instil this principle early on.

5. *What response has medical education made to the growth of psychiatry?*

Some, but little enough. The days when all this subject required seemed to be satisfied by four or six visits to a mental hospital, where the superintendent would put some bizarre psychotic patients through their paces, are past, though not long past. Nowadays teaching hospitals have flourishing departments of psychiatry with a reasonable allotment of in-patient beds. Three months of the student's last clinical year is usually shared between psychiatry and some other specialty and during it he will often spend one or two weeks living in a mental hospital or working in a psychiatric unit at some other general hospital.

But is this enough for a subject that is involved, it is sometimes claimed, in up to 30% of the cases a general practitioner will see, a specialty that is the biggest outside general medicine and surgery, and which, moreover, embraces 40% of the hospital beds in the country? Few teaching hospitals, it is safe to say, cope with all the psychiatric problems that occur in their neighbourhoods and fewer still teach their students either to watch for emotional components in patients with ordinary diseases, or emphasise how complex is psychiatry as practised in the community.

6. *Have teaching hospitals adapted themselves to an ageing population—and to the fact that an increased proportion of all disease is now in old people?*

Again, hardly at all. It has long been difficult to secure the admission of aged patients to teaching hospitals. The general view has been that they are not "good teaching material" and that by their tardy progress they block beds. The specialty of geriatric medicine has therefore grown up independently of the teaching hospitals and is still largely ignored by them. Informed instruction about the special complexity of aged patients, their liability to have many diseases and

[1] *Report of the Royal Commission on Medical Education.*

disabilities simultaneously, to suffer furthermore from both psychiatric and social handicaps, is a field from which the medical student is excluded. This is his loss, for, whether he ultimately works in general practice or as a non-teaching hospital physician, psychiatrist, specialist in community medicine or as an orthopaedic surgeon, he will spend an increasing part of his time with the old and must learn for himself what he has not been taught.

It is true that many London teaching hospitals are in the process of expanding to engulf other hospitals in their neighbourhood and that these other hospitals have often already set up geriatric units and appointed geriatric physicians. Students may pay occasional visits; in some areas they may be seconded there for a week or a fortnight. But the subject remains peripheral, an appendage to the curriculum like forensic medicine, not part of the main track. The contrast with the other end of life could hardly be greater. Here the decline of infectious disease has given paediatric teachers the opportunity, grasped almost everywhere, to extend the range of their teaching, to impress on their students the relevance of social and psychiatric factors in many of the remaining disorders of childhood, and the importance of prevention.

For very much the same reason teaching hospitals tend to exclude patients with chronic diseases—not entirely, of course, but the tendency is there. It is true that the distortion of a student's experience by the exclusion of such cases from the wards is to a large extent compensated for by his encountering them in the out-patient clinic. But his stint is limited. He may see a patient at intervals over a period of three or six months—only a fragment of time in a disease such as rheumatoid arthritis or schizophrenia, ulcerative colitis or hypertension, which may trouble and disable a patient for ten, twenty or thirty years. Has the capacity of film to telescope time yet been exploited in teaching about chronic disease?

7. *Is the need for postgraduate pre-registration medical education being satisfied?*

Here the answer is even less flattering. Most people agree that the introduction of the compulsory pre-registration year in Britain in 1953 was sound in conception. It is often very unsatisfactory in practice. Posts may be held in small hospitals with poor laboratory and library facilities, where the clinical material has little variety, where teaching hardly exists, and where the shortage of other doctors entails too long hours of duty and too little time for study—the pair-of-hands problem. These unsatisfactory posts are by no means exceptional as was found in a survey published in 1964.[1] It is high time that the universities should undertake a continuing responsibility for this period of training.

If, and it is a large if, the recommendations contained in the two latest and weightiest reports[2][3] are carried out the answers to all these seven questions may be quite different in a few years' time. In addition, post-registration postgraduate training will have been transformed. It will no longer be, to quote *The Lancet*[4], "little short of chaos"—and the most important reason for the steady stream of British-trained doctors crossing the Atlantic to Canada and the United States and crossing the world to Australia will have evaporated.

All these plans hinge upon money and resources being found to train more doctors. So long as the present shortage continues postgraduate training schemes, refresher courses and specialty training for general practice will be pie-in-the-sky. And Britain cannot expect to staff the lower ranks of its hospital service indefinitely with graduates from overseas who are badly needed by their own countries. Indeed, the doctor shortage is world-wide. The United States, aware of its dependence on graduates trained overseas, has thirteen more medical schools in the process of formation in addition to the fifteen new ones already open; Norway already trains half its medical undergraduates overseas and is to open a third medical school in the north;[5] France has a need for twice the present number of medical students:[6] Sweden plans to increase its doctors-per-million population from 1,040 to 1,430 by 1980;[7] in 1965 nine Commonwealth countries in Africa had fewer than 100 doctors per million population.

Allowing for no change in the emigration/immigration balance the Royal Commission on Medical Education suggests that the intake of British medical schools should be doubled over the next twenty years. Unless this is achieved the quality of postgraduate training is bound to suffer. So will the quality of medical services available to the public.

These medical services, the context of medicine, are our next concern.

---

[1] Hutton, P. W., Williams, P. O., Graves, J. C. and Graves, V. (1964), *Lancet*, **i**, 38.
[2] *Recommendations as to Basic Medical Education.* General Medical Council.
[3] *Report of the Royal Commission on Medical Education.*
[4] *Lancet*, (1966), **ii**, 1399.
[5] Harlem, O. K. (1968), *Brit. Med. J.*, **i**, 441.
[6] Mensh, I. M. (1967), *J. Med. Educ.*, **42**, 1101.
[7] *Report of the Royal Commission on Medical Education.*

CHAPTER TWELVE

The Framework For Practice

In the first chapter of this book medicine was compared to a mobile: a mobile of five pieces—disease, patient, doctor, their relationship and the context in which medicine is practised—the movement of any one of which alters the whole. Later chapters have given some instances of how the medical mobile can be set dancing. New diseases, the new patients who contract them and the new patients who have no disease at all—these have profoundly jolted the doctor component of the mobile from his old static position; and in the last chapter he was shown to be totally unprepared by his education and training for the new demands that are constantly being made on his services.

In this chapter the fifth component of the mobile will be discussed, the context in which medicine is practised. One country after another has abandoned, or greatly modified, the old individual direct patient-doctor relationship based on the payment of a fee at the time of illness. The rising cost of scientific medicine is making the prepayment of fees and the other expenses of treatment necessary except for the very rich. But there is still plenty of scope for argument about the best method of prepayment: taxation, compulsory insurance, voluntary insurance, or a combination of them. How each country has decided in favour of one form of prepayment rather than another depends on such things as national history and prevailing political philosophy. So, again, it is the British example that is dealt with in detail, partly because Britain's national health service has aroused more controversy than the more limited schemes of other Western countries, and partly because the historical background of all these other schemes, without which they cannot properly be appraised, could not be given within the scope of this book.

The Effect of the English Poor Law

There are many dates that could be chosen as the starting point of

Britain's health service. Most people perhaps would see its origins in Lloyd George's National Insurance Act of 1911, which by means of compulsory insurance provided Britain's workers, below a certain income, with the services of a doctor as well as a weekly payment during periods off work because of sickness. Others would trace the health service to the great sanitary measures and the setting up of a short-lived Board of Health that sprang from the cholera and other epidemics of the nineteenth century. But if only to emphasise at the outset that the predominant influence determining the shape of Britain's health service was the Poor Law, perhaps the best date to take is 1834.

This was the year of the Poor Law Amendment Act and the introduction of the principle of "less eligibility". The relief of the poor in their own homes (known as "outdoor relief") had become too costly; the poor, according to the prevailing philosophy, were poor through their own fault; they could not, of course, be allowed to starve to death, but at least they should be maintained only in such degrading circumstances that their fellows would not be tempted "to quit the less eligible class of labourers and enter the more eligible class of paupers". Arthur Hugh Clough's lines

> "Thou shalt not kill; but needst not strive
> Officiously to keep alive:"

so often wrongly quoted in support of euthanasia—or at least of allowing the very old and the suffering to die in peace—were in fact a scathing indictment of Victorian hypocrisy such as was exemplified in the prevailing attitude towards the relief of the poor. This attitude led to the building of huge brick workhouses and infirmaries, many of which still stand today as its visible legacy, and which, together with the large asylums that were the fruit of the Lunatics Act of 1845, have become part of the health service's capital stock. In the nineteenth century the sheer horror of workhouse life, coupled with the stigma of pauperism and the loss of civil rights which it imposed on those driven to it, made, as an American historian[1] has pointed out, "the welfare state inevitable by the end of the century. A system of public relief deliberately made hideous for its recipients could not long outlast the grant of universal franchise".

The sick poor were not intended to be treated as paupers and forced to enter the workhouse along with the able-bodied poor. They

---

[1] Gilbert, B. B. *The Evolution of National Insurance in Great Britain: The Origins of the Welfare State.* (Joseph. London, 1966), p. 15.

were still to be allowed outdoor relief, and if they had to leave home they ought, according to the Poor Law commissioners, to be housed in buildings set up specially for them. But the elected boards of guardians, whose duty it was to administer the new policy, found that even if they wanted to make a distinction between the sick and the able-bodied, it was often not possible. Moreover, outdoor relief for the sick was thought to encourage malingering so that the work-house test was imposed in cases of doubt; and the small fixed payment made to the Poor Law doctor for attending all the sick poor of the district encouraged him to have them admitted to the work-house as soon as possible. When they were admitted it was not to separate establishments; these did not exist because they would have been too expensive to build and maintain.

Thus, thirty years after the Poor Law Amendment Act some 50,000[1] sick people had accumulated in the workhouses. At the same time the sick who should have been removed from the community—because they were suffering from the deadly infectious illnesses of the nineteenth century—might be refused admission on the ground that they were dangerous.

In 1867, after the appalling condition of the sick in the workhouses had been brought to light through private and official investigations, the Metropolitan Asylums Board was set up to combine the Poor Law districts for the purpose of building isolation hospitals for infectious illnesses. More important was the provision in this legislation that gave the Poor Law Board power, backed by the weapon of finance, to insist that the guardians, or combinations of them, should start or adapt hospitals for the sick poor. The obligation of the state to provide hospitals for the poor, a task that had hitherto been left to charity through the voluntary hospitals, had been recognised.[2]

Even now, not very many of them were built either in London or in the provinces, to which similar, though less effective, legislation was applied in 1868–69. The short era of enlightenment, during which a genuine attempt was made by the central authority to remove the sick from the stigma of pauperism, did not last long. On the establishment of the Local Government Board in 1871, the man who was appointed permanent secretary was John Lambert, a strong believer in the deterrent principle of the Poor Law. Once again, the policy pursued was to curtail outdoor relief in favour of institutional relief, and though Lambert wanted this institutional provision to

---

[1] Abel-Smith, B. *The Hospitals* 1800–1948. (Heinemann. London, 1964), p. 49.
[2] Ibid., p. 82.

be separate from the workhouse it still carried with it the taint of pauperism. In addition, his influence was predominant in the Local Government Board as a whole. John Simon, who brought with him, when he and his assistants were transferred from the Privy Council, an enthusiasm for preventive medicine by means of improved sanitation and the notification of infectious illness, was pushed into the background. Had this not happened, had the public health zeal of Simon been able to combine with the attempts of Lambert's predecessors to set up dispensaries and hospitals that, though within the Poor Law, lacked its deterrent aspects, England would have gone some way towards a national health service in the 1870s.

As it was, although a class of non-pauper patients gradually found its way into the Poor Law hospitals and infirmaries and although after 1885 the stigma of disfranchisement was removed, the public hospital system of Britain was still a Poor Law system down to 1930. Not only did this make "the welfare state inevitable". More important still in the context of the growth of the country's health services all measures of social reform from the turn of the century had to be divorced from the Poor Law if they were to be acceptable to the new philanthropists—the Barnetts and the Webbs—and to the emerging Labour party.[1]

Moreover, the Boer War had shown up the poor condition of the army's recruits. The Victorian belief in the virtues of a free market for labour, which a deterrent Poor Law was intended to strengthen, had been shown up as an illusion. The workers whom the free labour market called forth were hardly strong enough to hold a gun.

Thus, for a short time at the beginning of this century, but not for the last time, the cause of national efficiency and the cause of humanitarianism went hand in hand.[2] An interdepartmental committee on physical deterioration confirmed the evidence of malnutrition and general unfitness that had already been produced by Charles Booth and Seebohm Rowntree. And among its recommendations were an adequate system of school medical inspection and the provision of school meals for needy children, not simply because it was inhumane to let children go hungry, but because if they were sick or hungry they could not take advantage of the education provided for them by the state.[3]

The school medical service, "for the first time, provided personal medical services on public charge entirely outside the jurisdiction of

---

[1] Gilbert, B. B., op. cit., p. 15.
[2] ibid., p. 60 ff.
[3] ibid., p. 123.

Q

the Poor Law authorities".[1] But the first real breach in the Poor Law had come two years earlier. In 1906 the Education (Provision of Meals) Act enabled local education authorities to feed hungry children and stipulated that if their parents could not, or even would not, pay the necessary charges, they were not to suffer the loss of civil rights that they would have done under the Poor Law. Historically, this was the beginning of Britain's welfare state.[2]

Although it excited far less public attention, in and out of Parliament, the plans for a school medical service immediately ran into complications. It was one thing to make the medical inspection of schoolchildren compulsory, but who was to treat the disease, defects and disabilities that inspection would disclose? This was a question that immediately concerned the principles and purses of doctors, and a committee of the British Medical Association set itself to find an answer.[3] Children might be treated under the Poor Law; but then either many parents would refuse and their children would go untreated, or, if the Poor Law taint were removed, so many parents might take advantage of this form of provision that the private doctor would suffer. The same consideration—the effect on the doctor's purse—would apply if children were sent to the voluntary hospitals to be treated by charity. Thus the only possible solution was the establishment of school clinics, which provoked the further question of how doctors were to be paid for their services in these clinics. Not surprisingly, with the prospect that clinics would prove an unpredictable burden on the rates, and faced by the pressure from doctors to restrict free treatment in clinics to the poor, the local authorities were at first reluctant to set them up, even when encouraged to do so by an act of 1909 that put the treatment of schoolchildren whose parents failed to pay for it outside the Poor Law on the same basis as had already been done for school meals. By the time clinics were being set up in any number, and the First World War was putting a stop to the Liberal party's social reforms, the doctors had fought and lost their battle with Lloyd George over national health insurance.

The act introducing old age pensions had become law on 1 August, 1908. They were to be paid to people aged seventy and over after a test of means. They were paid from public funds, but with the stipulation that no one receiving them would lose his civil rights. But old

[1] Eckstein, H. *The English Health Service.* (Harvard University Press. U.S.A. Oxford University Press. London, 1959), p. 19.
[2] Gilbert, B. B., op. cit., p. 102.
[3] ibid., p. 149 ff.

age pensions were the last of the big social reforms of the prewar years through which the Liberal government deliberately attempted to break up the Poor Law by the provision of relief for particular classes of people, and particular needs, through agencies outside it. This relief did not preclude a test of means to establish that it was needed—though in the case of school meals and the treatment of schoolchildren parents who refused to pay generally escaped penalty and in any case were not pauperised. But in seeking to extend pensions, to provide maintenance for widows and orphans and for the sick and the unemployed, Lloyd George and Churchill introduced an entirely new principle into Britain's social policy, the principle of social insurance, which was imported straight from Germany.

The Lloyd George Scheme

The working man, for whom national health insurance was soon to be compulsory, already contributed small sums in one way or another to provide himself with medical treatment and sick pay. There were medical clubs, to which patients might pay as little as a penny a week to obtain the services of a doctor. There were provident dispensaries for the same purpose. Above all, there were the friendly societies, which, together with the industrial insurance companies,[1] formed the first barrier to Lloyd George's scheme. The friendly societies flourished in nineteenth century Britain as a voluntary alternative to the poor law. But by the end of the century, because of the great fall in mortality resulting from higher standards of living, public health measures and the defeat of a few of the great infectious diseases such as cholera and typhus, they were in grave financial difficulties.[2] Their members were not dying in their former numbers. Instead they were living on until old age and its consequent infirmities overtook them, and the friendly societies found themselves paying pensions in the form of sickness payments. Thus the societies raised no objection to the grant of old age pensions by the state because these would reduce their liabilities to the old. National health insurance for the working population was a different matter; it threatened their very existence. Similarly the industrial insurance companies objected strongly and successfully to Lloyd George's

[1] Industrial insurance companies might be limited liability companies like the Prudential. Or they might technically be friendly societies if they were registered under the Friendly Societies Act of 1896 to obtain tax exemption. But industrial insurance, of either type, was distinguished from the true friendly societies by being a profit-making industry, by restricting benefits to payments at death and, especially, by sending agents at frequent —probably weekly—intervals to people's homes to collect the premiums.
[2] Gilbert, B. B., op. cit., p. 170 ff.

original proposal to include widows and orphans in his scheme because, unlike the true friendly societies, the companies normally provided death benefit only—they made large profits out of their customers' abhorrence of a pauper's funeral. Any payment by the state to a breadwinner's dependants the companies identified with a payment following death and therefore regarded as inimical to their interests.

There is no need here to go through Lloyd George's tortuous and intricate dealings, first with the friendly societies and then with the industrial insurance companies. Put simply, he had a battle to fight on three fronts and he chose his tactics accordingly. First, he proposed to give the societies a privileged position in the administration of his scheme. Then he enabled the industrial insurance companies to take part on the same terms. This renewed the hostility of the friendly societies; for they knew that they would not be able to compete for national health insurance members on equal terms with companies that sent agents every week into people's houses to collect premiums for death benefit. But the insurance industry was Lloyd George's most powerful opponent. By winning over its support he felt strong enough to meet his third enemy—the medical profession. Thirty-five years later, another Welshman dealt similarly with opposition to the proposed national health service. By offering in 1946–48 the consultants and specialists employment in the service's hospitals on favourable terms Aneurin Bevan was able to meet the hostility of the general practitioners.

In 1911, as had happened before and was to happen later, the doctors' spokesmen were to pay lip service to the principle of a better form of medical care, while objecting to almost every means by which the principle was to be put into practice. Indeed, at this time the American Medical Association seems to have been more forward-looking than its British counterpart. While the British Medical Association was trying to consolidate the opposition of its members to Lloyd George's bill, the *Journal of the American Medical Association* was publishing articles in support of it; the culmination was a leading article in its issue of 23 November, 1912, which said that although the act was "probably the most revolutionary, so far as medical practice is concerned, of any measure yet introduced in an English speaking country, the controversy between the Government and the physicians has been almost entirely over the question of compensation and not over the principles on which the act is based". Approving the new position of the doctor, "working for the general good rather than as a private, professional or business man", the *Journal* commented that similar arrangements "will, sooner or later, be considered on this side of the Atlantic".[1] That it was more than fifty years before a similar measure became law in America, and then only in the teeth of the most vehement opposition from the American Medical Association, shows how very far advanced the views of its *Journal* were in 1912.

But it was not entirely correct in assuming that the only difference between the Government and the profession was one of money. The doctors were rightly concerned about their position *vis-à-vis* the friendly societies. Under the old arrangement they were regarded by a society as custodian of its funds and expected to control malingering. Friendly societies rarely permitted free choice of doctor, because if doctors were dependent upon their patients' good will for their income, they would be more likely to give them certificates of sickness. So the doctors were under contract to the friendly societies, and the members of a society had to accept the doctor who was appointed to look after them. Two of the British Medical Association's "six cardinal demands", announced before the bill became law, were free choice of doctor and the removal of medical benefits—in effect, the living of doctors—from the hands of the friendly societies. This demand Lloyd George met by an amendment that set up insurance committees, which were to establish a "panel" of doctors joining the scheme from which the prospective patient would choose his own.

But the real weapon that Lloyd George used to defeat the doctors was money. The main vocal medical opposition to his scheme came, not from the humble general practitioners who would run it, but from the physicians and surgeons of the great voluntary hospitals, probably provoked by fear that national health insurance would reduce the contributions made by friendly societies to the hospitals' funds. The general practitioner, on the other hand, was badly paid; how badly neither the Government nor his association realised until an investigation showed that in five towns his average earnings were 4s. 5d. a patient a year. Another of the British Medical Association's cardinal demands was adequate payment, defined as 8s. 6d. a head, excluding the cost of drugs. By increasing the proposed capitation fee to 9s. including drugs, less than three months before the scheme was due to come into full operation, Lloyd George was guaranteeing doctors who joined it an income of 7s. a patient, an increase of almost 60% on what they were getting. By the time Lloyd George was explaining to the Insurance Advisory Committee early in 1913 how the Government proposed to counter the British Medical Associa-

[1] Quoted by Brand, J. L. in *Doctors and the State*. (Oxford University Press. London, 1966. Johns Hopkins Press. U.S.A., 1965).

tion's boycott,[1] 11,000 doctors had already joined the panels. Within a week nearly 15,000 had done so.[2]

Medical Planning between the Wars

Lloyd George certainly never intended the national health insurance scheme to be bounded by the act of 1911. Its two main deficiencies were the lack of any cover for the dependants of the insured and the lack of any institutional cover for anyone—with the exception of sanatorium treatment for the tuberculous insured. With the establishment of the Ministry of Health in 1919, a council on medical and administrative services was set up under the chairmanship of a well-known doctor, who later became Lord Dawson of Penn. He had already, a year previously, voiced his personal view that curative and preventive medical services should be undertaken together in specially equipped centres, a view that was echoed by an advisory committee of the Labour party,[3] with Beatrice Webb on it, at about the same time. Now Lord Dawson was to produce a truly radical report.[4] His council recommended the establishment of primary health centres, staffed by general practitioners but visited by consultants, which would have beds for the in-patient treatment of simple cases and which would also house the preventive services. Other more serious or complicated cases would be referred to the secondary health centre, which in effect would be a hospital. Unlike the Labour party's advisory committee, the Dawson Report did not envisage a full-time salaried service for doctors, nor did it recommend that general practitioners should abandon their own private surgeries for consultations. But the centre was intended to bring them and senior hospital staffs together, to break down the compartmentalisation of the profession and to serve as a focus for its interests; in other words, to do what the medical centres set up in district hospitals over forty years later are intended to do.

Some of the members of the council considered that the service should be entirely financed from public funds. Most thought that the patient should pay something towards its cost, but doubted whether,

---

[1] In effect, it was proposed to engage doctors on a fixed salary; this would have pleased the friendly societies as more likely to prevent malingering, and they would therefore have been encouraged to give these doctors a monopoly both of insurance practice and of private practice among the families of the insured.

[2] Gilbert, B. B., op. cit., p. 415.

[3] The Labour Party. Memoranda prepared by the advisory committe on public health. *The Organisation of the Preventative and Curative Medical Services and Hospital and Laboratory Systems under a Ministry of Health.* (London, 1918).

[4] Consultative Council on Medical and Allied Services. *Interim Report on the Future Provision of Medical and Allied Services.* (H.M.S.O. Cmd 693. 1920).

as a rule, he could make more than a contribution. The principle behind the council's recommendations, which also included the co-ordination of public and voluntary hospitals, was that "the organisation of medicine has become insufficient and ... fails to bring the advantages of medical knowledge adequately within reach of the people."

The Dawson Report had a favourable reception in the press and even, to begin with, from the British Medical Association. But the impetus to reform, born of the war, was soon lost. The report was written and published during the postwar boom, when England was still expected to become a land fit for heroes. It was also a time when the rising prices accompanying the boom intensified the difficulties of the voluntary hospitals. In spite of new sources of income in the form of payments by public authorities for services rendered (the treatment of venereal disease, for instance, and of tuberculosis, which was removed from national health insurance in 1920), the voluntary hospitals entered the inter-war years on the verge of financial collapse and had to be helped by a grant from the state. By the time this salvage operation had been carried out, the postwar boom had collapsed; the fall in wages and prices enabled the voluntary hospitals to carry on without further public aid; and the notorious Geddes Committee on government expenditure, the Geddes axe, in 1922 effectively stopped any more spending on health—the first Minister of Health, Dr Addison, who had been one of the parliamentary architects of the 1911 act, had already been dropped by Lloyd George a year earlier after an outcry against allegedly extravagant spending on local authority housing.

So the next twenty years were to be a period not of expanding and extending Britain's embryonic health service, nor of bringing together its two hospital systems, but of plans and reports discussing the pros and cons of doing so. However, one piece of legislation of great significance was carried through. This was the Local Government Act of 1929. It enabled the local authorities, through health committees of the counties and county boroughs, to provide general hospitals outside the Poor Law either by new building or by converting the workhouse infirmaries. By the time the Second World War broke out the number of beds in local authority hospitals (excluding Poor Law infirmaries) nearly equalled the number in voluntary hospitals. The voluntary hospitals were no longer the only form of institutional provision for the ordinary sick to be without the stigma of the Poor Law.

Of the reports and recommendations that were published in these inter-war years, three should be mentioned. A Royal Commission on National Health Insurance,[1] which reported in 1926, recommended its extension to the dependants of the insured and the introduction of a specialist out-patient (though not in-patient) and domiciliary service through the insurance scheme. Much more far-reaching proposals were to come from the official Committee on Scottish Health Services[2] (the Cathcart Committee), which reported in 1936. Echoing the report of the Royal Commission on Health Insurance, it envisaged a "unified" health service, in which the general practitioner, as family doctor, would have been the linchpin. He would have been in independent contract with the local authority, which would have had the duty of providing the services of a general practitioner to all people needing them who were outside the insurance scheme. Because the same authority was also responsible for environmental and preventive health services and, since 1930, for hospitals, the family doctor would no longer have been working in isolation from these other branches of medicine. Moreover, the voluntary hospitals were to have been co-ordinated with the municipal hospitals to prevent overlapping and to allow scarce beds to be used to the best advantage. Here, in fact, was a blueprint for an ideal health service. Because it was so ambitious, the report provoked a powerfully argued reservation,[3] which foresaw, if the report's recommendations were carried out, the introduction of a state medical service financed out of rates and taxes. "The pernicious habit of getting something for nothing will be encouraged, which is bound to have a detrimental effect on the morale of the people."

A year after the Cathcart Committee reported, Political and Economic Planning, an independent research body, produced a report[4] on the health services. Less ambitious and idealistic than the Cathcart Committee, it nevertheless exposed very clearly the existing defects of the system of medical care in Britain from the point of view of the consumer. "The voluntary hospital system has made it hard to arrange to assign patients to the hospital which can best treat them, and in many cases the size of the hospital or its range of functions are not such as to secure the most efficient working . . . One of the great weaknesses of the [local authority] system is its dependence upon local government areas rarely, if ever, corresponding with the most natural and efficient region which the hospitals, if untrammelled,

[1] *Royal Commission on National Health Insurance.* (H.M.S.O. Cmd. 2596, 1926).
[2] *Committee on Scottish Health Services.* (H.M.S.O. Cmd. 5204, 1936).
[3] Sir Andrew Grierson. *Reservation regarding the proposed extended general practitioner service.* Cmd. 5204.
[4] *Report on the British Health Services.* PEP.(London, 1937).

would serve. Almost everywhere the needs of patients and of hospital efficiency are cut across to varying degrees by arbitrary administrative boundaries and by lack of adequate reciprocal arrangements."[1] As for the general practitioners, to whom PEP, like the Cathcart Committee, allocated a key role in the medical care and health education of the family, they "are rarely able in existing circumstances to fill the role thus marked out for them". "The panel doctor . . . often has neither the facilities nor the equipment which, as precise diagnosis becomes daily more possible, are necessary to provide an adequate service. As a result he passes on his patients to the hospital . . . and often enough he tends to become little more than an agent for signing certificates . . . Instead of his medical and intellectual interests being stimulated by constant co-operation with members of the profession, as occurs in hospital practice, they tend to wilt in the solitude of general practice."[2] An extension of national health insurance to cover consultant services would, PEP thought, bring the general practitioner into stimulating contact with the consultants.

But if, as PEP also recommended, the insurance scheme were extended to the dependants of the insured and to others in similar economic circumstances (that is, with incomes of less than £250 a year or, say, £20 a week now), the total insured population would be about doubled at 38 million, or 85% of the population of Great Britain. Clearly such an extension might impose an intolerable burden on panel practice unless it were made more efficient, and the way in which greater efficiency could be achieved would be the replacement of the individual isolated practitioner by "a small team of doctors . . . having at their disposal diagnostic apparatus and premises which no one of them could afford to maintain . . . it seems likely that the position of general practitioners could be very much strengthened, and public confidence in them fully restored, if they could evolve some acceptable system of working in local groups from well-equipped central dispensaries."[3]

Thus, at the beginning of the Second World War, Britain's health services had been planned several times over, and with a remarkable consistency between the proposals put forward. From the minority report in 1909 of the Poor Law Royal Commission onwards, the emphasis had been on the need for a unified service, the importance of preventive medicine, the anomaly of two hospital services, and

[1] Ibid., p. 17.
[2] Ibid., pp. 162–3.
[3] PEP: p. 164.

the end of individual isolated general practice concerned solely with curing disease. Over the years, too, the philosophy behind reform had become clearer. In contrast to the Webbs and other Fabians, and indeed to the medical officers of health, Lloyd George did not think of the national health insurance scheme as a means of providing the British working man with a system of medical care outside the Poor Law. To him it was a scheme, like old age pensions, for the relief of poverty.[1] If the breadwinner were sick, he and his dependants might be pauperised, so he ought to be guaranteed some income during his illness. The treatment of his illness was an afterthought to the income benefits, and it did not have to be extended to dependants' illnesses because, as non-workers, they did not contribute to the family income.[2] To the Webbs and their fellow-thinkers, on the other hand, sickness was as great an evil as poverty. Because people were poor, they were sick; but outside the Poor Law, with all its deterrent characteristics, they could not be provided with the means to get better. Therefore there should be a unified medical service, based on health committees of the larger local authorities, which would also take over the public hospitals, and through this service people should be virtually bullied into living healthy lives and benefiting from the progress of medical science.

From the idea that people ought to take advantage of the progress of medical science, it was a short step to argue that they had the right to. Thus in 1918 Mrs Webb was asserting through the Labour party's advisory committee on public health[3] that; "Disease is no respecter of persons, and science in dealing with its prevention and cure cannot afford to be so", and that: "Modern methods of diagnosis and treatment are becoming so elaborate and costly that only the rich can afford to purchase their advantages . . . Many a patient has lost his life through trying to save a doctor's bill," Similarly the Dawson Report,[4] two years later, noted "the increasing conviction that the best means of maintaining health and curing disease should be made available to all citizens". Throughout the twenties and thirties it came to be taken for granted that a health service was justifiable in its own right; it did not need the *raison d'être* of relief of poverty. The argument was restricted to ways and means. Should the service be taken out of social insurance and be provided out of public funds— the "ultimate solution" propounded by the Royal Commission on National Health Insurance (although it did not recommend it at the

---

[1] Gilbert, B. B. op. cit., p. 314 f.
[2] Gilbert, B. B. op. cit., p. 314. Also Cmd. 5204, pp. 21–2.
[3] Labour Party. Memoranda. 1918.
[4] Cmd. 693, 1920.

time) and by a minority of the Cathcart Committee? Or should health insurance be extended to cover 85% of the population (as suggested by PEP), with the uninsured of low income covered by the public assistance medical service—in effect, the Poor Law as renamed by the Local Government Act of 1929—and the wealthier making their own arrangements as before?

But the individual need was also seen as the common good. Just as the report of the Committee on Physical Deterioration, confirming the poor physique of British soldiers in the Boer War, provided the right climate of opinion for the introduction of school meals and the school medical service, so the condition of recruits in the two World Wars was attributed among other things to the inadequacy of medical care. Thus in 1918 the Labour party's advisory committee contended: "Health is of national concern, and disease is a national danger, hence the health of every individual, rich or poor, is of national importance, and its preservation should be undertaken by the nation collectively."[1] In 1936, the Cathcart Committee referred[2] to the "conscious concern for the quality of the race" that, mingled with other motives, had been behind the expansion of the public health services. A few years later, the publicity given to the head lice, impetigo, scabies and bedwetting of many of the young evacuees from city slums[3] echoed the outcry provoked by the condition of the Boer War recruits.

From the contention that health is of national concern it was easy to argue that the nation would benefit if it spent more money on the promotion of health and the prevention and treatment of disease. Against this extra expenditure should be set the gain to the community from fitter workers. Health meant wealth, and "we cannot afford not to have it" became the password that opened every door to Britain's welfare state.

From Beveridge to Bevan

In this context the Beveridge Report,[4] which late in 1942 assumed a comprehensive health and rehabilitation service as a necessary part of a social security scheme, though separately administered, was not strikingly radical. Indeed, the doctors themselves had gone almost as far earlier in the same year. The draft interim report of the British Medical Association's medical planning commission envisaged a

[1] Labour Party. Memoranda. 1918.
[2] Cmd. 5204, p. 25.
[3] *Our Towns: a close up.* (Oxford University Press. London, 1943).
[4] *Social Insurance and Allied Services.* Report by Sir William Beveridge. Cmd. 6404.

comprehensive health service, based on regional authorities, for 90% of the population; the general practitioners would work from health centres, which would also house some of the public health services; and the consultants would have either whole-time or part-time salaried posts in the hospitals. These recommendations, which went far beyond the British Medical Association's previous attempts, in the thirties, at planning a health service, were endorsed at its annual representative meeting, with the significant modification, carried by a bare majority, that provision should be made for the whole community instead of 90%, but with patients having the right to contract out. There were doctors favouring even more radical proposals than the medical planning commission's, notably a group calling itself Medical Planning Research, whose plan for a comprehensive free service was published shortly before the Beveridge Report. The significant point is that when Beveridge signed his report, he knew that the doctors were not opposed in principle to his Assumption B (the establishment of a comprehensive health service), in contrast to their attitude towards Lloyd George's much more modest scheme of 1911.

It was not just the doctors who were not opposed to the idea. It would have been hard in 1942–45 to find anyone in Britain who would have questioned the need for a health service. Even PEP, which in 1937 had firmly said that the "state of public finances would not permit" a free health service comparable to the educational service, was urging by 1944 that the proposed service should be available to all who wanted it, not merely to the 90% of the population who were less well off, for "medical needs may be unlimited, while incomes never are". What Mr Attlee was to call (and his choice of words was significant) "not just a glorified Poor Law, but a full health service for all the people" seemed, in the later years of the war, to follow as naturally as the night the day.

But the ways and means of providing a health service still had to be decided. A choice had to be made between three forms of organisation: first, extended national health insurance, with bigger contributions to cover the bigger benefits; second, putting the whole cost on to the taxpayer and ratepayer; third, charging the patient, according to his means, at the time of his using the service: or a combination of all three forms could have been adopted. The drawback of the first method was that in Britain national health insurance had become identified with the approved societies that ran it, and the disadvantages of the approved societies had been shown up more than once. It was the approved societies associated with industrial life insurance that had the largest membership—nearly half of all those compulsorily insured in 1938—and industrial insurance had acquired a bad name through its salesmanship methods and its high administrative costs. Further, the approved societies, whether associated with industrial insurance, friendly societies or trade unions, gave widely varying additional benefits—additional, that is, to the statutory payments during sickness and the services of a doctor. These benefits were paid out of any surpluses the societies might realise at periodic valuations. Thus, the insured in a high risk industry, who most needed things like hospital and specialist treatment or surgical appliances, were the least likely to get them.

It was still possible, of course, for the health service to be paid for by compulsory insurance, but without the agency of the approved societies. But the Beveridge Report recommended otherwise. First, its plan for social security assumed (the famous Assumption B) that comprehensive health and rehabilitation services would be available as a corollary both to payments by the state of high benefits during sickness and to the receipt of these payments by individual citizens, who "should recognise the duty to be well and to co-operate in all steps which may lead to diagnosis of disease in early stages when it can be prevented"—an echo of the Webbs and the minority report on the Poor Law. The assumption would not be fully realised if the availability of the services depended upon insurance contributions. Secondly, the Beveridge plan recommended a flat rate contribution from all those in the social security scheme because contributions and benefits related to earnings would not have provided a subsistence income for those with low earnings when they were out of work, through sickness or unemployment, or retired. Had an extra contribution towards the cost of a health service been added to the flat rate contribution for social security payments, the total would have been too heavy for low incomes to bear.

Nevertheless part of the proceeds of the national insurance contribution was allocated, in accordance with the Beveridge recommendations, towards the cost of the health service; and it is worth noting that in the first official plan for the service, published in 1944, this contribution was intended to cover as much as 27% of the total. In actual fact the proportion covered by insurance was never so high even as 20% simply because of the serious miscalculation of the service's probable total cost. It has since fallen to about 11%, in spite of periodic increases in the amount of the contribution.

If entitlement to health service benefits through insurance was to be ruled out, it was still open to the Government to charge the cost of the service to public funds but to impose charges on patients at the time of using it. This would not, after all, have been remarkable. When local authorities were enabled, under the Local Government Act of 1929, to build general hospitals, they were required to charge patients according to their ability to pay. Voluntary hospitals, though originally established to give the poor a free service, were charging patients by the outbreak of the Second World War, and a great many private hospital insurance plans had emerged to meet the fees. Why, then, did both Churchill's and Attlee's governments decide to dispense with patients' payments altogether?

Part of the answer lay in the existence of about 21 million people already receiving free general practitioner treatment and free drugs through the national health insurance scheme. They could hardly be asked to start paying. Apart from this practical difficulty, there was a lingering suspicion in the Labour party, voiced[1] as long ago as 1922, that so far as the voluntary hospitals were concerned he who paid most got a favoured and speedier service. Any continuance of preferential treatment for the better off was felt to be particularly intolerable during a war when equality of sacrifice was asked for and when "fair shares" of food, coal and other rationed commodities was a ruling principle. Then, again, the exigencies of war had already entitled sections of the population to free services.[2] Evacuated children, for instance, were given free treatment by general practitioners and in hospital. So were air-raid casualties, internees and, for a short time, the aged and infirm found living in air-raid shelters or miserably trying to maintain a bare existence at home. Where services were not free the local authorities had the unenviable task of recovering contributions from, say, evacuated mothers, who might not stay with them long, and then trying to obtain the balance of the cost from the mothers' own normal local authorities, under the old Poor Law rules, or from the Ministry of Health if they were evacuees under an official scheme. So complicated[3] were the financial transactions between one local authority and another, and between the authorities and the ministry, and so little was yielded, by comparison with time spent and clerks employed, from charges to the beneficiaries of the services, that it is not surprising that the Government decided that the collection of payments from patients was more trouble than it was worth.

[1] Trades Union Congress and Labour Party. *The Labour Movement and the Hospital Crisis.* (1922).
[2] Titmuss, R. M.: *History of the Second World War: Problems of Social Policy.* (H.M.S.O. London, 1950). pp. 227–279, 467–470.
[3] Ibid. Chapter XII passim. p. 469.

Lastly, any such collection had to be made according to a patient's means. Before the war local authorities had developed their own means tests for deciding how much anyone should pay for hospital care, and these tests were not stringent. But if there were to be a national health service, there would have to be a national means test to determine ability to pay for it, and the first experience the country had had of a national means test was the notorious test for unemployment relief first introduced in 1931. "Means tests," said PEP in its report on Britain's Health Services in 1937, "have become odious"—a grave understatement. In its short life (in 1940 it was replaced by a milder test of needs and applied to the old as well as the unemployed) the household means test, which penalised the thrifty unemployed and the working members of their families, did more damage to the Labour party's emotions than almost any other social measure. It was the old Poor Law again but writ very large indeed, for it applied not to a comparatively few unemployable but to a million or more unemployed who genuinely wanted work. But unlike the disfranchised paupers of the nineteenth century the unemployed retained the vote. Any Labour government that was to represent them would find it very hard indeed to include a means test in such an emotional service as the treatment of the sick.

This account of the origins of Britain's health service is too cursory. Its intention is to show that the service's gestation lasted for at least a generation and in some senses for over a century; the British people did not demand one simply as a postwar treat for having fought the Second World War from beginning to end. A comprehensive health service, free at the time of use, was a logical outcome of planning and experience, not something suddenly brought forward by a starry-eyed Labour government tasting effective power for the first time. Has it succeeded in what it was intended to do? Or ought the exercise never to have been attempted?

Perhaps the first thing that should be said is that most people in Britain approve of the health service.[1] Any idea that they are gravely disillusioned and critical of its working is greatly exaggerated. A Swiss journalist, coming to London in 1964 after an absence of many years, said that he had only one question to ask about the health service: why was it that Britain had had thirteen years of

---

[1] See, for instance:
Institute of Economic Affairs. *Choice in Welfare* 1965. Appendix A.
Cartwright, A. *Patients and their Doctors: a study of general practice.* (Routledge and Kegan Paul. London, 1967). p. 217.
New Society, 19 October, 1967.

Conservative government and not abolished it? The answer was equally simple: no Conservative government wanted to, and if it had wanted to, it would not have dared to. But because over the years its stresses and strains have become apparent, and are now given more attention than its successes, it is worth while to draw up a balance sheet.

Advantages of Britain's Health Service

The hospital system constitutes the most important and tangible benefit provided by the health service. One has to go back to look at the utter confusion in Britain's hospital service before 1948 to appreciate what has since been achieved—or, rather, hospital services, for there were two separately administered, overlapping, types of hospital, the voluntary and the local authority. The growth of the latter, from its Poor Law origins down to 1930 when the larger authorities were enabled to establish general hospitals outside the Poor Law, has already been outlined. But in the same hundred years the voluntary hospitals were also changing. By the beginning of this century the advance of medical science had already led to a demand for voluntary hospital beds from patients willing to pay, just as there was a growing class of non-pauper patients in the Poor Law infirmaries. By the twenties and thirties hospital contributory schemes were flourishing and providing the voluntary hospitals with an independent source of finance. At the same time a typical voluntary hospital had ceased to be a great teaching hospital, with unpaid senior doctors who used their hospital appointment as a permitted form of advertisement to attract rich patients to their Harley Street consulting rooms. It was just as likely to be a so-called cottage hospital of, say, thirty to a hundred beds where general practitioners treated their middle class patients. The consequence of the haphazard growth of the voluntary hospitals and the connection, just beginning to be broken down, between the public hospitals and the Poor Law was that in 1939 there were beds all over the place but a true consultant medical staff only in areas where there was a rich enough private practice to sustain it and where one or two enlightened local authorities, notably Middlesex, broke away from the normal hierarchical structure of public hospital staffing and employed consultants on a basis of equal status and responsibility. There was also a difference of function between the two systems. The voluntary hospitals tried to restrict their admissions to acute cases, who would not block much-needed beds. The public hospitals could not select their cases and therefore tended to have large numbers of their beds filled with the chronic sick and the elderly.

At the outbreak of war in 1939, therefore, the Ministry of Health, wanting to make plans for dealing with the expected hordes of air-raid casualties, found itself faced with two hospital systems that were hardly anywhere co-ordinated and whose staffs and managers were not disposed to co-operate with each other. On these two systems the Emergency Hospital Scheme had a far-reaching effect. At the expense of the ordinary civilian sick, many of whom were discharged prematurely from hospital or refused admission, the Ministry of Health imposed something like a unified system on the hospitals through linking them together for medical purposes irrespective of which system they belonged to and irrespective of local government boundaries. Originally intended to provide solely for civilian and service casualties of war, the emergency scheme, when the air-raid victims turned out to be so very much fewer than had been estimated, became responsible for sick soldiers and eventually, when the ordinary needs of civilians could be denied no longer, for many of them as well. Further, in order to provide adequately for casualties the Ministry of Health up-graded many of the hospitals by supplying them with operating theatres and essential facilities like X-ray departments; it also provided about 50,000 new beds.[1]

There was, during most of the war years, no government intention to abolish the voluntary hospital system. Even in 1944, the first white paper[2] on a national health service envisaged the voluntary hospitals as having a contractual relationship with the proposed joint local authorities that were to provide a hospital service. But wartime experience showed up the weakness of the dual system. The voluntary hospitals, paid by the central government to keep beds free for casualties, were not disposed to reopen beds for the treatment of the civilian sick because this would have meant losing some of their subsidy. The effect was an extra pressure on the public hospitals' beds and complaints of staffs being overworked in those hospitals while others were underemployed.[3]

Furthermore, by the end of the war the Ministry of Health had found itself closely involved in the running of the hospitals in a way it had not foreseen.[4] It was concerned in the recruitment and pay of nurses and with patients' food. It employed consultants and organised their distribution. It introduced a rehabilitation service for the

[1] *A National Health Service.* Cmd. 6502. (1944).
[2] Ibid.
[3] Titmuss, R. op. cit., p. 454.
[4] Ibid. p. 482, 503.

R

injured and national laboratory and blood transfusion services. It received complaints from patients about the quality of the services rendered. The decision to have one national hospital system instead of two systems in uneasy relationship with one another was logical.

The only real alternative was to nationalise the voluntary hospitals and hand them over to the local authorities. There were several reasons for rejecting this solution. The local authorities, whose finances before the war were inadequate for many of their functions, now had to face the obligations of the 1944 Education Act and heavy expenditure on housing. They could not have taken on a hospital service as well. Even had they been able to, local government boundaries were usually quite inappropriate for a service that needed to transcend them, partly because a hospital's natural catchment area did not correspond with them and partly because some specialist services needed an area much bigger than that of most local authorities to be used economically. That problem might perhaps have been solved by the proposals for joint authorities in the 1944 white paper. But there remained the reluctance of voluntary hospital medical staffs to be employed in a local authority service. The reluctance sprang from the old association of the local authority hospitals with the Poor Law, from their obligation to take any case submitted and their consequent overloading with—in doctor's eyes—the less interesting chronic sick, and from their hierarchical staffing structure, with the top salaries going to the medical superintendent, an administrator not a clinician. Doctors were also afraid of local authority interference in clinical matters. And there were more imponderable things like name and status to be taken into account. The board and staff of Guy's Hospital would never have agreed to become subordinate to the London County Council. As it was, the teaching hospitals, in London and the provinces, were allowed to retain their endowments and some of their independence.

There can be endless argument about the actual organisation of the new hospital service, about whether the doctors had too much say in running it, about whether too much responsibility was given to the regional boards and too little to the management committees of the individual hospital groups, about whether the Ministry of Health interfered too much or was too passive in the early years when the service was taking shape, about whether the English teaching hospitals should have been integrated into the regional plans as they were in Scotland. But that Mr Aneurin Bevan, as the postwar Labour Government's first Minister of Health, was right to set up a single hospital system based on regional divisions rather than on local government boundaries has never been seriously questioned.

Aneurin Bevan's decision to nationalise the hospitals and set up a single hospital system relieved the consultants of their anxiety about becoming employees of local authorities. Whereas in 1911–12 it was the members of the royal colleges who openly opposed Lloyd George (see page 245), in 1946–48, with the promise of payment for their hospital work and the right to retain private practice they were easily attracted into the health service. It is the duty of the Minister of Health under the National Health Service Act of 1946 (and this is the second advantage of the health service) to provide specialist facilities throughout the country; their availability is no longer determined by which side of a local government boundary a patient lives on or by whether a voluntary hospital happens to be in the right place and happens to provide the necessary specialist cover.

PEP's prewar report gave a figure of 221,345 beds in voluntary and public hospitals combined in England and Wales in 1935–36, excluding hospitals for mental illness, subnormality and infectious diseases. About 1,866,000 in-patients were treated. Thirty years later, with only about 30,000 more beds available, the hospitals treated 4,574,000 in-patients. Or, to make a statistical comparison between 1949—the first complete year of the health service—and 1967, in the latter year in all types of hospital over 5 million patients (2 million of them surgical cases) were treated in a total of 467,447 beds. In 1949, 2,937,000 patients were treated in 453,000 beds. This improvement in hospital efficiency is by no means exclusive to Britain; but at least it shows that in this respect the health service has not failed.

The figures reflect not only a better supply of specialist skill but also a bigger demand for it. One reason for the bigger demand is the removal of the financial barrier, which brings us to the third advantage of Britain's health service, the fact that it is free at the time of use.

On medical grounds it is clearly better that a condition should be treated early rather than late, and if a patient does not have to find the cost, or part of the cost, of treatment he is more likely to seek it early. The application of science to medicine has made the cost of treatment rise dramatically and therefore made the problem of paying for it more urgent. Moreover, medical needs are unpredictable, and a patient electing to enter hospital cannot be certain of knowing the total cost of treatment in advance.

The absence of all fees and payments makes it much easier for a doctor to recommend and carry out whatever he thinks necessary for the patient's recovery. So the fourth advantage of Britain's health service is the freedom of the doctor. By this is meant freedom from financial transactions with patients, freedom to exercise his professional skill without asking himself whether a patient can pay for it or whether he should pass the patient on to a less skilled but cheaper colleague or whether he should act charitably. The absence of these considerations adds to the self-respect of both doctor and patient.

Further, the doctor no longer has to worry about whether his bills will be paid. The financial security which doctors enjoy is another advantage of Britain's health service. Despite periodic complaints and threats of strikes British doctors have not, as a rule, been underpaid by comparison with other professional people with incomes guaranteed by the state. General practitioners' earnings vary according to the work they do; many of them earn as much as a university professor. A wholetime consultant with an A merit award[1] earned £9,275 a year in 1969, and fees for visits to patients' homes might bring him another £924. At the top a wholetime consultant can earn as much as a top rank civil servant. Hospital staff below the rank of consultant began, as house officers in their pre-registration year, at £1,250, and in their last training grade as senior registrars were paid £2,760 a year at their maximum.

Doctors' real complaints, though often expressed in terms of pay, are about overwork and conditions of work. These complaints highlight the disadvantages of the health service.

Disadvantage of Britain's Health Service

The first disadvantage of Britain's health service is that it rested on a fallacy—the fallacy that if medical care were more readily available to more people ill-health would be reduced and that a healthier population would make the country richer. On the contrary, the provision of any form of medical care always makes sickness more overt, and the danger facing any government embarking on an extension is that sickness becomes too overt. Has Britain reached that point?

Complaints of over-use are constantly made; and one reason for the suggestion frequently made by doctors that the patient should pay something at the time of using the service is the wish to check

[1] In addition to their salaries about one in three of consultants (part-time or whole-time) receives a merit or distinction award. These were distributed as follows in 1969, the part-time staff receiving a *pro rata* amount:
100 A Plus awards of £5,275   1,030 B awards of £2,350
340 A awards of £4,000   2,110 C awards of £1,000

excessive and unnecessary demand. They have a case. But there is evidence that over-use is not noticeably greater than in countries where fees are paid.[1] In Britain the average number of consultations given by a general practitioner is five per patient a year. In America a comparable figure is 4·5; among countries with compulsory insurance, where fees are subsequently reimbursed in whole or part from an insurance fund, the Federal Republic of Germany is one with a much higher rate (over ten), and only Sweden among the countries surveyed had a much lower one, probably because it has comparatively few doctors in relation to the population. Nothing definite emerges from any such comparisons except that the payment of a fee is only one variable among many determining the demands on a doctor's services.

And what constitutes over-use? Attendance at a doctor's surgery with a complaint of headache? Or three days in a private ward in a hospital for a check-up? Judged by the demands made on the total medical resources of a country, the first, though free at time of use, costs less. One suspects that in Britain, as elsewhere, doctors feel differently about over-use or unnecessary use of their services according to whether their patients are private or not.

Money, or rather the lack of money, is one of the handicaps of the health service. Hospital waiting lists could be reduced, and over-crowded surgeries relieved, if enough money were spent on the health service to produce more beds and operating theatres and to attract more doctors. The grave disadvantage of a health service dependent so largely on public funds is that it has to compete with other claims on the national purse, particularly, in the social sphere, with schools and housing. This disadvantage is especially apparent in postwar Britain because it has been subject to so many economic crises, all of which have been met by the imposition of cuts, or at least ceilings, on Government spending.

The reluctance to spend money on new hospitals is notorious. Britain's health service was in the unfortunate position of having inherited in 1948 a stock of old buildings that though lamentable by the standards of twenty years later, and even considered pretty poor at the time,[2] were at least serviceable. Had this stock not existed in 1948, the Government would have been compelled to allocate more money to hospital building—or to reject the whole notion of a national health service.

---

[1] Cartwright, A. op. cit., p. 25, quoting from Logan et al., *National Centre for Health Statistics* (U.S.A.) and Weber, *Some Characteristics of Mortality and Morbidity in Europe.*
[2] *Hospital Survey Reports.* (H.M.S.O. London, 1945).

The deliberate restraints put upon expenditure on the health service are illustrated in the international comparison made by Professor Abel-Smith for the World Health Organisation.

TABLE 9

TOTAL EXPENDITURE ON HEALTH SERVICES
(CAPITAL AND CURRENT)
AS PERCENTAGE OF GROSS NATIONAL PRODUCT

Country	Year	as % of GNP
Israel	1961/62	6·3
Canada	1961	6·0
United States	1961/62	5·8
Chile	1961	5·6
Sweden	1962	5·4
Australia	1960/61	5·2
Yugoslavia	1961	5·0
Finland	1961	4·8
Netherlands	1963	4·8
France	—	4·4
United Kingdom	1961/62	4·2
Federation of Rhodesia and Nyasaland	1960/61	4·2
Ceylon	1957/58	4·0
Poland	1961	3·7
Czechoslovakia	1961	3·6
Kenya	1961/62	3·5
Tanganyika	1961/62	2·5

Source: An International Study of Health Expenditure. B. Abel-Smith. Public Health Papers. W.H.O. Geneva. 1967. Table 24.

The United Kingdom ranks low among the advanced countries in the proportion of its gross national product allocated to health services. On the other hand Professor Abel-Smith enters a caveat about the conclusions to be drawn from any such comparisons. For one thing, a high expenditure on health services was found not to be related to medical needs as commonly recognised. Thus, the poor countries, with endemic disease and malnutrition, might because of their poverty spend comparatively little on the means of over-coming them. At the other extreme the United States, with a comparatively high expenditure, also had, and still has, a comparatively high infant mortality rate: in 1967 it was about 22 per 1,000 live births, compared with about 18 in England and Wales.

For another thing a high proportion of the gross national product spent on health services may merely mean that doctors have much higher incomes than other professional people or professional people as a whole than the rest of a country's inhabitants. Countries with a high proportion thus do not necessarily have a greater number of doctors for a given number of the population. In fact, from the same study, it appears that Czechoslovakia, with a low proportion of its gross national product spent on health, has more doctors (18) per 10,000 of the population than the United States (12·9).

But obviously if doctors' incomes are lower than they could earn in other countries, and at the same time emigration is freely permitted, doctors will be tempted to leave the health service. Doctors' earnings in Britain are not, as has been shown, low by comparison with those of other professions from which the element of risk has been eliminated. But if they are discontented on other grounds the high earnings of their colleagues elsewhere provide a big incentive to emigration. So the next disadvantage of Britain's health service is the discontent of doctors, which usually means the discontent of general practitioners and to a lesser, but growing, extent of junior hospital doctors.

It is hard to measure the success or failure of the general medical service because there are no yardsticks. Certainly, the health service, in spite of the controls on practice in overdoctored areas (the so-called "negative direction" of doctors), has not entirely rectified the maldistribution of general practitioners, though it has had some effect. The increase in out-patient consultations at the hospitals (1,575,000 more new patients seen in 1965 than in 1949) may be an indication of a genuine growth in the need for consultant advice on behalf of patients, or it may reflect the eagerness of busy general practitioners to shed some of their load.

This is an aspect of over-use that needs more attention. When general practitioners over-use the hospital service on behalf of their patients, by referring them to hospital unnecessarily, they encroach both on the time available to consultants for training junior staff and on the juniors' own time for studying and attending postgraduate courses. The consequent scamping of training for would-be specialists is an important cause of the brain drain.

The tendency on the part of general practitioners to act as "disposal agents"[1] also reflects the tendency on the part of their patients to regard them merely as "disposal agents", so glamorous has hospital

[1] E. J. Maude: *Reservation to report of Committee on the Cost of the National Health Service* 1956. Cmd. 9663, paras. 18–23.

medicine become, partly because of its actual achievements and partly because of its presentation on television in documentary and fictional form. For a hundred years the general practitioner has been gradually displaced from hospital medicine, as specialties developed and their practitioners expected exclusive control over hospital beds and admissions.[1] The health service was not, as so often alleged, responsible for this exclusion of general practitioners from the hospitals. But the service's structure encouraged it; moreover, the nationalisation of the hospitals took away from general practitioners their cottage hospitals, many of which had been built in the twenties and thirties to provide them with the beds and other facilities that they were denied in bigger hospitals. This divorce between the general medical and hospital services, which reflects the split in the medical profession, is another disadvantage of Britain's health service.

It is not merely the general practitioner and the hospital doctor who are divorced from each other. The local authority health services, concerned with preventive medicine and after-care, are divorced from both of them. Yet as long ago as 1920 the Dawson Report said that: "Preventive and curative medicine cannot be separated on any sound principle, and in any scheme of medical services must be brought together in close co-ordination. They must likewise be both brought within the sphere of the general practitioners whose duties should embrace the work of communal as well as individual medicine."[2]

Ideally the local health authorities and the general medical service should work together, with the doctor using the local health and welfare services to keep people out of hospital. The National Health Service Act envisaged co-operation by imposing on local authorities the duty to set up health centres. Until recently financial stringency and doctors' suspicions of local authority control have combined to prevent all but a handful of centres from being built. But there are now signs of a revival of interest and that general practitioners, in search of an identity, are coming to look more favourably on the importance of preventive medicine. Also, although administratively the health service is split into three parts, functionally it is drawing together. The attachment by some local authorities of nurses and health visitors to general practices, the increasing interest of the hospitals in illness outside their gates, the appointment of general

[1] Stevens, R. *Medical Practice in Modern England*. (Yale University Press. London, 1966). pp. 31–3.
[2] Cmd. 693.

practitioners as medical assistants in hospitals, and the growth of community psychiatry and geriatrics—all these trends are bringing the three branches of the medical profession closer together than this century has hitherto seen them. Late in 1968 the Minister of Health published a green paper intended to crystallise discussion on how they could best be drawn together administratively. To a large extent, however, reform must wait upon the reform of local government, which is also under review.

The building of new towns ought to give more scope to the integrated planning of the health services in them. There also seems no reason, apart from intra-professional restrictiveness, why there should not be more work for general practitioners in hospitals, especially for those who prefer hospital work to preventive medicine. This does not mean that they should perform work beyond their competence or training, as they tended to do in the cottage hospitals. But many medical cases are admitted to hospital who could be as well cared for there by their general practitioner, with consultant advice, as by a harassed junior hospital doctor. Such work would also make it easier for the GPs to retain the specialty that they are most reluctant to abandon—midwifery.

To sum up: the health service in Britain has neither created the problem of the right role for the general practitioner nor solved it. But the service, and national health insurance before it, have kept general practice alive as general practice. In the United States it has tended to disappear, at least in the cities where anyone who has a coronary attack may well be first attended to by a fireman; in other countries, for instance Australia, the general practitioner may undertake work that would be regarded as beyond his competence in Britain. But there too the trend is for hospital work by general practitioners to be eroded by the growth of consultant practice; before long Australia may therefore not be so attractive to emigrating British doctors as it has been. What is still not clear is whether the British taxpayer is keeping alive a branch of medicine that ought to be allowed to die. The answer is probably that the more specialist the rest of medicine gets the more necessary it is for the patient to have someone who, besides being a "primary physician"[1] and an expert in diagnosis, can also give advice, allay fears and educate. That there is a demand for such a doctor is shown by the popularity of doctors' columns in the press, particularly in women's journals, where fictional doctors give readers the health education that they ought to be receiving from the health service, and by the vast amount of

[1] McWhinney, I. R. (1967), *Lancet.* **i**, 91.

requests for medical advice that such papers receive.[1] In America, too, there has been discussion on how, not whether, the general practitioner can be revived.

Experience of Other Countries

Are the disadvantages of Britain's health service peculiar to it or have we anything to learn from other developed countries? Russia goes farther than Britain in having an integrated service, based on fully specialised hospitals at the centre, with polyclinics (a cross between out-patient departments and health centres) attached, and, in rural areas, clinics and health centres at the periphery, which strongly emphasises preventive medicine and health education. The organisation is very much like that planned in the Dawson Report of 1920, and the importance given to health education would have been approved by Beatrice Webb in 1909. Russian doctors are salaried employees of the state, and at least half of them are women. In Britain, medicine is still largely a man's preserve, but some at least of the shortage of doctors could be made good if it were made easier for married women doctors to stay in practice or to return to it.

In the rest of Europe, health services tend to be part of social security schemes and paid for largely out of insurance contributions from employees and employers. A common pattern is for the patient to pay first and then get back later either the full fee or a large part of it. This form of payment, it is argued, provides a deterrent to over-use of the service without causing hardship to those who genuinely need treatment. Further, it is also argued that the payment of a fee makes for a better relationship between doctor and patient. The latter argument is obviously not true in education of teachers and taught, and, in medicine, one wonders how much British doctors who advance it are only hankering after what they think was a golden age for British medicine. Nor has the patient's obligation to pay first and recover the cost later prevented France's health scheme from running into financial difficulties.[2] Indeed, the cost of the French service is comparable to Britain's, and French hospital building has also lagged behind the demands of modern medicine. If the disadvantages of Britain's health service largely spring from the method of paying for it, to replace taxes and rates by insurance contributions does not appear likely to overcome them. Nor has the insurance principle prevented doctors in one country after another from striking or at

[1] *Lancet.* (1967), **i**, 1205 and 1227.
[2] *The Economist.* 26 August, 1967. pp. 715–6.

least threatening to strike. Nor again have other systems of health care, any more than Britain's, been able to ensure that the expensive fruits of medical science, for instance haemodialysis and transplants, are available to all who need them.

Ought, then, the exercise never to have been attempted? Was the American Medical Association right in fighting to the last ditch the "Medicare" scheme for old people in the United States? Previously the United States had a dual standard of medical care for the population as a whole: a largely private medical market, covered by private insurance schemes, and a public service, like Britain's before 1948, for the poor and for those unable to buy medical care privately. (The Federal government provides medical care for members of the armed forces, veterans, merchant seamen and other small sections of the population.) Although the private sector is largely covered by insurance—perhaps, to some extent, because it is covered by insurance—the cost of medical care in the United States has risen astronomically. Between 1958 and 1967 the consumer price index (all items) rose by 16%. The total medical care index rose by 37%, but within that item the hospitals' daily service charge doubled.[1] So long as a rise in cost in hospital care can be covered by a corresponding rise in insurance there seems to be no limit that can be placed on it. And the more the average person has to pay in insuring himself against the cost of hospital treatment, the more he is likely to demand such treatment instead of asking for treatment at home from his doctor—whose fees he has probably not insured against.[2] That is one reason why the Medicare legislation allows old people extended care in a nursing, or convalescent, home after they leave hospital, and includes an optional scheme under which an old person can recover four-fifths of doctors' fees and other medical services.

In the long run, however, the most far-reaching part of the Medicare legislation may be Medicaid: federal grants to states that introduce approved schemes of care for the under-65s who are "medically indigent"—that is, cannot afford to pay for their own medical and hospital costs. The definition of "afford" is decided by individual states: New York's first definition, which allowed a family of four, with two earners, to be deemed indigent if their net income did not exceed £2,450 a year, was scaled down, but it is still the most generous. Other states have been more cautious. Even so,

---

[1] *Statistical Abstract of the United States* 1968. U.S. Department of Commerce. Bureau of the Census.

[2] Simpson, J. et al. *Custom and Practice in Medical Care.* (Oxford University Press. London, 1968). pp. 83–5.

the bastions of free enterprise medicine have clearly been under-mined.

These brief references to the financing of medical care in other countries seem to show that no country has solved the problem of how it should be done. The Russian system is the most logical on paper; but its advantages and disadvantages cannot be evaluated because neither patients nor doctors can freely voice their dissatisfaction with it. At the other extreme, the free enterprise system of the United States has produced such high costs that it has led to its own undoing.

On the other hand, where British medicine has something to learn from the United States, and other countries as well, is in its intra-professional organisation, as distinct from the organisation of medical services. From about the middle of the nineteenth century British general practitioners battled with the staffs of the voluntary hospitals, especially the hospitals specialising in particular diseases, whom they accused of treating, free, patients rich enough to pay general practi-tioners. From this struggle was evolved, around the turn of the century, the referral system,[1] by which specialists agreed not norm-ally to see patients unless they were referred by a general practitioner —though the restriction did not apply when a patient had no general practitioner or could not afford one. This practice can be justified as in the interests of the patient, who would otherwise have to decide for himself which specialist he needed. It can also be justified as an economical use of medical services, for a hospital's facilities are an expensive way of dealing with most of the complaints now diagnosed and treated entirely by a general practitioner—though probably many patients, without one, would sometimes not seek medical advice at all, and be none the worse for it.

But, however justifiable within the context of Britain's health service, which allows everyone the services of a general practitioner, the referral system is nevertheless a restrictive practice that would surely break down if patients had to pay their doctor for a referral to hospital. And if it broke down, or is frowned on by the Monopolies Commission in its present review of professional practices, where would the general practitioner stand? He might disappear altogether, or he might continue to practise in the community but be allowed to follow his patient into hospital. Thus the end of the referral system might just possibly end one general practitioner grievance.

Secondly, there are the demarcation lines drawn among hospital medical staffs. One—probably the main—reason why young doctors

[1] Stevens, R. op. cit., pp. 32–3.

emigrate is the lack of certainty about their future when they have completed their specialist training. Such a doctor, who has spent, after qualifying, six or seven years as house officer, registrar and senior registrar, has to wait until a consultant post in his specialty is advertised, and only if he is accepted for it can he be recognised and paid as a consultant. This insecurity drives doctors abroad, particularly to North America and Australia, where highly paid posts are available. If doctors who completed their training satisfactorily were assured of a well paid permanent hospital post, with the prospect of reaching full seniority after a certain age, Britain's hospital staffing problem would be greatly relieved. But the British medical profession has insisted on hospital doctors being either junior doctors in training or full consultants, with all the panoply of beds in their exclusive control and junior doctors under them. The profession's leaders are reluctant to abandon demarcation rules for fear that they would thereby allow a dilution of specialists; yet at the same time they deplore the hospitals' dependence on overseas doctors to make good the losses caused by emigration. They have confused the necessary and justifiable protection of the public through the imposition of high standards with the normal professional tendency to protect their own positions and pockets. One of the many sound recommendations of the Royal Commission on Medical Education is intended to enable a hospital doctor who has completed a specialist training to be classed as a specialist and to be a full independent member of a clinical team, even though he is not immediately appointed or paid as a consultant.

Perhaps there is also a lesson in this comparison of British and American medicine for those who argue that the exercise of trying to provide a health service should not be attempted, that medicine is a consumer's market which should be allowed the free play of market forces. The British health service, they assert, by its very nature prevents the expansion of facilities to meet the demand for them. If they were left to consumer choice they would increase to meet it—doctors, hospital beds and all. Yet the United States has had precisely this market. There, and in Canada too, doctors are big business and are among the wealthiest of the country's citizens. But the system does not produce enough doctors to satisfy the demand, and about a quarter of each year's addition to America's medical manpower comes from immigrants. The experience of the United States, even had Medicare not intervened as a reaction to high medical costs, surely suggests that, with the apparently unending march of medical science, there is virtually no limit to the number of doctors wanted. So long as there is money to pay for it, medical research has no bounds, and the number of doctors needed, to carry out research and ordinary medical care, has no limits either. It remains to be seen whether, now that federal funds are committed to an unknown extent in implementing Medicare, there will be a contraction in research spending. As it is, medicine as an international currency is hoarded in America like gold in Fort Knox. The high incomes and good facilities for doctors attract them from countries like Britain. Britain, as a consequence, has relied on attracting doctors who come for postgraduate training from the underdeveloped countries, which need every doctor they can lay hands on to carry out the preventive medicine programmes that ought to be the first concern of their embryonic health services. To complete the circle they receive some medical aid from the West. But the medical balance of payments is very much in the United States' favour.

Such experience as there is of a market in medical care does not, therefore, endorse the view that an extension of private medical practice on a big scale should be encouraged in Britain to expand facilities. To set standards, and to allow patients as it were a second opinion, a measure of private practice is certainly desirable and is appreciated by many doctors and patients. But the drawback of handing medicine over wholly or even largely to market forces is that the consumer of it does not have a free choice. He obviously does not choose to have appendicitis or pneumonia or schizophrenia. He does not choose, but relies on his doctor to advise, whether he should have this, that or the other drug for his complaint. On the other hand, there is a point, or rather a broad frontier, where medical care ceases to be a necessity and is a luxury, or at least what would be considered a luxury by many people. A system of care that allows a considerable amount of private practice would satisfy this luxury element to the detriment of the rest. Varicose veins, for instance, can be a disabling condition needing medical attention. They can also be merely disfiguring. A free enterprise medical system, financed from private insurance schemes, would allow surgeons to earn high incomes by performing operations on the varicose veins of every other woman over forty. But who, as a result, would have time to operate on the hernias of the labourers?

Perhaps the clash between medicine as a luxury and medicine as a necessity can be best seen in mental illness. In the United States psychiatric practice is most profitable in the psychoanalysis of patients who can afford it. The consequent flow of psychiatrists to treat neurotics, and those who want an analysis as a form of consumer spending, has not helped the plight of the mentally ill in the state mental hospitals, where in 1964 29 out of 279 had no psychiatrists on their staff at all.[1] If the improved distribution of medical resources to the mental hospitals has been one clear gain from Britain's health service, the American private enterprise system is in this respect shown at its greatest disadvantage. In both countries, of course, public opinion and medical opinion is far from content with the amount of resources devoted to the care of the mentally ill. In the United States, informed opinion, stimulated by a report of the Joint Commission on Mental Illness and Health, is more vocal than in Britain and has the backing of the Federal government, which through the National Institute of Mental Health provides grants to states for setting up psychiatric units in general hospitals, for more community care and for the education and training of staff. Psychiatrists in Britain envy the training programmes in the United States; but neither as regards psychiatrists nor as regards nurses and social workers can America apparently overcome the obvious deficiencies in its mental hospitals, where the daily cost of care is between a sixth and a seventh of the cost in general hospitals (compared with about one-third in Britain), and at the same time satisfy the demands of private practice. In the fifteen years up to 1964 neither the proportion of the national income spent on psychiatry, nor the amount of the state budgets allocated to it, increased. The psychiatric example does not justify the contention of right-wing liberal economists that to allow more private practice would, by increasing the total resources available, in the long run improve the standard of health service practice. In the short run, simply because private patients demand more time and personal attention from their doctor—which are what they are paying for—any encouragement of private practice is bound to encroach on the needs of the health service.

This is the real dilemma facing doctors, whatever the form of medical care that their particular country has adopted. There are clearly recognisable medical needs—illnesses or ill-health—that everyone agrees should be met, whether by a publicly provided service or by private enterprise. Beyond these needs there is a seemingly unlimited demand for doctors' services that has been generated by the advance of medical science, and by the mass media that have publicised it. There is also a demand that has been provoked by a wider definition of needs, especially by the increasing pervasiveness of psychiatry: what appears to be an unjustified demand today

[1] Canada: Royal Commission on Health Services. *Trends in Psychiatric Care* by McKerracher, D. G., 1964.

becomes tomorrow's need. It would be tempting to say that the role of a state service should be to cover needs only, as the Poor Law was intended to do, and that demands should be met by private practice and private insurance. But this would be an over-simplified solution: first, because of the tendency, apparent in the United States, for needs to be submerged by demands; secondly, because an individual doctor, faced with an individual patient, may find himself uncovering a real need presented as an unnecessary demand, irrespective of how his services are being paid for in the particular case. The reverse can also be true: what began as a clear expression of need can be extended to unnecessary demands.

The medical mobile is set moving by this interaction of demands and needs; but it cannot be said that one form of the medical care under which the interaction takes place is more likely than another to determine the mobile's new resting position in favour of the doctor. The only certain conclusion is that, in distinguishing needs and demands, and justifiable demands from—in the existing context— unjustifiable ones, a doctor must have imagination as well as a scientific training.

Epilogue

"I should never have been happy in any profession that did not call forth the highest intellectual strain, and yet keep me in good warm contact with my neighbours. There is nothing like the medical profession for that: one can have the exclusive scientific life that touches the distance and befriend the old fogies in the parish too . . ."

Middlemarch.

Nearly a hundred years ago, through the mouth of Tertius Lydgate, George Eliot proclaimed what, broadly reinterpreted, has remained the ideal of most young medical students. But is this ideal still valid? Or have the processes at work in this century forced doctors to choose between the two sides to their profession: the scientist and the artist? Are the two cultures ineradicably opposed? Has the ascendancy of scientific medicine, which in the care of the astronauts has enabled specialists to touch a distance that Mr Lydgate never dreamed of, left the general doctor searching for a role? Progress in science, as has been shown in so many of the previous chapters, has created new problems while solving others: problems for the profession and practice of medicine; problems of economic and social policy; and ethical problems that society has barely begun to appreciate, let alone to solve.

This final chapter seems to be the right place to bring together these strands from earlier parts of the book and to try to weave them into the pattern that this century presents. The pattern contains other strands, many of them science-based, but many not. Surprisingly, there are few that do not have some connection with medicine, even if this link is tenuous, circuitous and tangential.

Science and the Practice of Medicine

The march of science has made it almost impossible to combine "the exclusive scientific life" with "good warm contact with my neighbours". "Befriending the old fogies", with the rise in numbers of the old and the decline of churchgoing, has largely become a job for professional and voluntary social workers. But the aged sick remain

8

with the geriatric physician and the generalist, two of the newest of the specialties (paradoxically, general practice is now regarded as one) into which medicine is all but fragmenting.

Moreover, the pace of change that science has dictated in medicine has illuminated the slowness of medical education to adapt itself. But there are signs that radical changes are in the wind.

The Economic and Social Consequences of Scientific Medicine

Most of the new advances have led to a large increase in the cost of medicine. Where a disease can be prevented by immunisation—poliomyelitis, for example—a medical discovery can be seen to save money as well as life or lifelong disablement. Where a drug, or a series of drugs, has been developed to treat a disease that formerly consumed a great deal of medical resources—for instance, tuberculosis—large savings are made. Most of the new developments in medicine, however, demand very much more money—money for machines, for laboratory work, money to pay for doctors' time and skill. This rise in cost inevitably reduces the time they can spend in, for example, seeing sick old fogies. Many of the recent advances in medicine concern treatment for common chronic diseases. Instead of dying soon patients with diabetes live for decades but continue to see their doctors, attend clinics, and become occasional in-patients; instead of staying inexpensively in a mental hospital for decades—cheaply, that is, in terms of doctors' time—schizophrenic patients who recover incompletely need follow-up appointments, visits from mental welfare workers, and not infrequently repeated readmission.

Two further developments in medicine have both increased its cost and contributed to the rising demand on doctors' time. First, modern medicine involves doctors in seeing well people. Immunisation clinics have to be staffed; doctors are expected to take part in family planning, in health education, and in giving genetic advice. The newer and developing topic of screening and its offshoot, the identification of the high-risk case, will employ still more of their time.

Secondly, the concept of disease has widened. Obesity, alcoholism itself rather than solely its neurological consequences, cosmetic surgery, and childhood behaviour disorders—to select only one of psychiatry's new preoccupations—are nowadays regarded as within medicine.

The newest growing points of medicine—renal dialysis units, organ transplantation, and intensive care and coronary care units—are notoriously costly in terms of both money and doctors' time.

These features of science-based medicine, and the almost unlimited demand for doctors' services (and the necessary equipment and ancillary staff) that they provoke, are common to all the advanced countries of the world. They ensure that nowhere, even in the most affluent societies, are there enough doctors. The United States cannot meet the demand from its own medical schools and pulls in British doctors, attracted as much by the facilities for postgraduate training and research as by the promise of a higher standard of living. In Britain, in turn, the necessity to staff a health service, on which demands never stop rising, conflicts with the needs of post-basic medical training. The gap is filled at present by graduates from underdeveloped countries. They too are attracted primarily by training facilities, but they stay on in larger numbers because the conditions of medical practice are so much more congenial than in their own countries. The circle is completed, as we have seen in the last chapter, by two links: American doctors—few in comparison—who help to implement medical aid programmes in Asia and Africa, programmes in the main concerned with environmental and preventive medicine; and British doctors, perhaps 1,600 in all, who are resident in developing countries, of whom 500 work in government medical services overseas.

In advanced countries these environmental and preventive services—clean water, adequate drains, immunisation—have long been provided from local and central funds. This century has seen the personal health costs of an individual, particularly the costs of his treatment in hospital, become increasingly a responsibility of central government. The steepness in the rise in cost of Western medicine is overwhelming the voluntary insurance principle, the main bastion against the erosion of private medicine, but other more secular forces have been at work. Mass-communication, for example, has ensured that huge numbers of people know of medicine's advances and demand the fruits; but, even more, the right to health, insofar as medical science can ensure it, has gradually come to be regarded as a basic human freedom, an extension of the century's pervasive egalitarianism, that none the less remains a right for being so patchily granted.

It is strange that the United States, where Roosevelt proclaimed his Four Freedoms and for a time the home of Thomas Paine who affirmed the Rights of Man, should have been so laggard in acknowledging this new right, which its scientists and doctors by their labours have done so much to give meaning to and to forward. To those who have no neurotic fears of "creeping socialism" Medicare and Medicaid, like the British health service, represent no more than moves towards, if not health, at least the treatment of disease in people whose societies have long granted the right to literacy and numeracy.

No end is in sight to the rocketing costs of medicine. Events in the last twenty years have amply proved the error of supposing that the devotion of ample resources to medicine would be a once-for-all investment that would lead in time to a fall in demand through improved health. The fact is that whatever is made available by technical advance in metropolitan centres—sophisticated surgery, kidney machines, intensive care units, coronary flying squads—will soon be demanded in towns and villages. In equity they can hardly be denied. But by now the costs of medical services compete with those of other publicly provided services, roads, education and the like, and the competition requires political decisions. However much doctors deplore the fact, medicine, because of its huge cost, is now in politics and bound to stay there.

Nor is the increasing demand for metropolitan medicine restricted to the advanced countries of the West. In developing countries the first step should be to concentrate on raising the standard of living, to check communicable disease, to provide environmental health services, and to advise on birth control. Doctors there need to be managers first, without any direct relationship with their patients, and personal physicians second.[1] But educated minorities in underdeveloped countries will insist on this personal medicine in the same way as they refuse to be fobbed off with other goods and services considered by aid planners to be more appropriate to their needs than the Western things they want. The scanty resources of these countries could easily be exhausted by the supply of high-cost Western medicine, while outside one or two towns the medical services resemble those in the Britain of more than a hundred years ago.

Is there any solution to the voracious and mounting demand for doctors' services? The conclusion of the previous chapter was that no country has yet found a way of providing medical care that satisfies both the patient–consumer and the doctor. So insatiable is the demand that resources have to be rationed: in a free enterprise country this will be effected through the purse; in countries like Britain the shortage shows in waiting lists with priority for the most seriously ill, and in the frustration and discontent of doctors. There is always danger, too, that excessive demand will lead to falling standards of medical practice.

[1] McDermott, W. (1966), *Amer. J. Psychiat.*, **122**, 1398.

One way, of course, to relieve the pressure is to dilute medical skill. There is nothing very new about this. Health visitors, laboratory technicians, physiotherapists, medical social workers (who can befriend the old fogy in the parish) all do work formerly done by doctors. This process could go and is going much farther. In Russia and elsewhere medical workers with shorter training carry out many of the tasks traditionally reserved in the West for graduates of the great medical schools. Even in Britain there is a move in general practice towards letting trained nurses sort out trivial conditions and deal with them. But there are many other fields where those with a much more limited training could carry out limited tasks: immunisation and vaccination; examining cervical smears; fitting coils; many screening procedures; and much of the work involved in haemodialysis.

Another way lies in installing more machinery, more automation in laboratories, in computer-assisted diagnosis, computer-suggested treatment schedules, and so forth. But there is a danger here. Fifty years ago the Labour party's advisory committee complained: "So much of the practitioner's time is spent on the art of medicine, in visiting, humouring, and encouraging his patients, that too little remains for acquiring and practising the science of medicine." Most people are now probably uneasy that the pendulum has swung too far the other way: that the results of scientific tests need interpreting; that powerful drugs must be used with discretion; that the basis of wise medicine remains a relationship and that no patient can relate to a computer. Too much of medicine must not be delegated. The old fogy must never be forgotten.

New Ethical Problems

In this century some ancient ethical problems of medicine have been given a new urgency by technical advances, by new or at least freshly realised social needs, or by broad trends of change in what society expects of its members. A reduced birthrate has made children more precious. At the same time wide acceptance of psychology and social science has convinced people that to be unwanted gives a child a poor start in life and is likely, moreover, to increase his chances of becoming delinquent, neurotic and, in turn, a poor parent. It is no surprise therefore to find that the legal grounds for *abortion* have been widened, so far in many places as to amount to social reasons alone.

The stern ban on *medical self-advertisement* is being eroded by the public thirst for information on health matters. While the press and the radio remained the chief sources from which this thirst could be quenched anonymity could be largely preserved, but the rise and triumph of television as the dominant medium have made the ban seem rather ridiculous. Unsigned articles are still part of an acceptable convention, and unidentified voices can speak with authority; but unnamed faces, perhaps because the face gives so many clues to personality, are merely irritating. Diehards in the profession may shake their heads in disapproval, but if medical authority has taken anyone to task for television publicity, the public has yet to hear of it.

As an ethical problem *contraception* has involved medicine late in the day when it had almost ceased to have moral aspects. Its steadily increasing use has been based essentially on the same changes in attitude as underlie the liberalisation of abortion laws: that children should be wanted and that an unwanted child is a threat to a family's economic and psychological security. Many of these arguments bring contraception within the boundaries of social medicine, particularly social psychiatry. Contraception has survived religious and social taboos and thrived; it has survived the demographic argument that it was wrong because it would result in a fall in the population; it has survived the social class argument that it is dysgenic; it has survived the strategic or imperial argument; and it has been proof against population projections that have time and again turned out to be wrong. In Britain it is now officially encouraged and, of course, in the world at large it is looked on as the foremost means of salvation from ultimate starvation. The Pope alone has not concurred.

Medicine has more recently become directly concerned because the cap, the coil and the Pill, the only contraceptive methods that have a failure rate of less than 10% (less than 10 failures per 100 woman years), need medical intervention. And medicine, therefore, has to concern itself with the sole remaining moral issue of contraception—the supply of advice, pills, devices to the unmarried, particularly the teenage population. Though some doctors may refuse to take part there can be little doubt about which way the issue will be settled. To a post-Freudian and post-Kinsey world an ostrich attitude to the facts of the sexual imperative, at its most imperious in late adolescence, will no longer do. These things happen whether society's elders approve or not. Perhaps they always did happen but were unacknowledged; perhaps social disapproval used to ensure silence and secrecy. Even if the moralists are right—and there is no evidence whatever that they are—that an increase in teenage sexual activity is a consequence of postwar permissiveness, of a general fall in moral standards, there is no social sense whatever in not safeguarding society against the consequences. The argument that the provision of sexual education and of contraceptive facilities for the young will encourage promiscuity is unproven.

Abortion, self-advertisement and contraception were ethical problems involving medicine before the Second World War. Many new ones have been thrown up by medicine's advances since then; so many, indeed, that it is impossible to deal with them in detail.

The controversy about *euthanasia* has been discussed in Chapter 6 in relation to the aged senile, grossly deformed children, those in severe pain from incurable cancer, and people with irreversible brain damage from road accidents. The dilemmas of *experimental medicine*—how far should experiments on human beings go? what safeguards should there be?—are dealt with in Chapter 2. In Chapter 2, also, some of the ethical difficulties in *renal dialysis* and *renal transplantation* have been mentioned. The appearance of heart transplants above the horizon has shown that when it comes to unpaired organs the ethical problems, if not the technical and immunity ones, are worse. If a beating heart is taken from a patient whose brain is irretrievably and totally damaged is this homicide? Will the law have to be altered so that legally tissues can be obtained immediately after death more easily than at present? The questions can be multiplied till they become tedious.

These are some of the problems that could keep doctors, lawyers, theologians and philosophers busy till the end of the century. One can reasonably echo Sir Derrick Dunlop: "It is often difficult not to be nostalgic for the days when social, political, and ethical problems facing our profession were not as formidable as they are now, and, when they did exist, were debated discreetly . . . within the profession."[1] Debate can inform and enlighten, but decision and responsibility in this unfamiliar and expanding field of non-therapeutic relationship ought to remain, as Sir Roger Ormrod has stressed,[2] firmly with the individual doctor.

The Future

If our civilisation survives into the next century, if it avoids the danger that world resources will be exhausted by a galloping crisis of overpopulation, if it avoids nuclear destruction and some less explosive decay caused by its own internal weaknesses, what are the preoccupations of medicine likely to be then? Such a forecast can

[1] Dunlop, D. reviewing *Medicine on Trial* by Dannie Abse (1968), *Brit. Med. J.* ii, 107.
[2] Ormrod, R. F. G. (1968), *Brit. Med. J.* ii, 7.

only be put forward in the most tentative fashion, an extrapolation, in essence, of trends that have developed over the past few decades.

At the start of such a dangerous discussion, as a corrective, the old error of reification must be remembered: disease is an abstraction; there are no diseases but only sick people. The question therefore needs rephrasing—at the end of the century what will people see doctors about?

1. It seems likely that the remaining infections, particularly the virus diseases, will be conquered, although—if some reification can in this instance be forgiven—they may fight many a rearguard action.

2. It is quite likely, too, that many of the problems of cancer will have been solved—a bold assertion, but justifiable on balance.

3. In this connection, it is probable that people will much more often visit doctors when they are well for the early detection of disease.

4. Chronic bronchitis, the English disease, should have yielded to preventive measures.

5. Psychiatry can be expected to have mastered the non-organic psychoses.

6. Whether gerontology and research into the causes of degenerative disease will have had many practical results is another matter, and much more doubtful. Spare-part surgery, especially if progress can be maintained in dealing with the immunological problems of rejection, may well have developed enormously to mitigate the results of degenerative disease.

7. Congenital malformations, inherited disease, metabolic disorders —this is another field in which great progress should have been made, preventive, corrective and palliative.

8. So far, so good. The predictions rest upon continued progress in physical science and in the more exact of the biological sciences— pharmacology, immunology, virology, radiology, genetics and bio-chemistry. There is no reason to doubt that this growth will continue to bear fruit. But any progress in dealing with the new diseases (Chapter 10), with neurosis and with behaviour disorders, demands from psychology and social science a firm base of established fact on which to build. So far these sciences have been unable to provide a corpus of knowledge, though lack of this has not prevented prag-matic treatments, such as behaviour therapy in some behaviour disorders and group therapy in alcoholism, from achieving some success; nor has it prevented society from handing over an increasing amount of delinquent behaviour to doctors for treatment because of the bankruptcy of penal methods.

But there is no sign in this field of a breakthrough comparable with the discovery of antibiotics or of the contraceptive pill. We lack the knowledge to answer the questions. What is addiction? If, as seems firmly established, smoking cigarettes is overwhelmingly the most important cause of cancer of the lung why do so many people still smoke cigarettes—and start to smoke? Of the majority of the population who drink alcohol why do some destroy themselves, and wreck their families, by excess? If taking too little exercise and eating and smoking too much are root causes of arterial disease and coronary attacks, why do so many people overeat, walk so little, and use their cars so much? Why do some people misuse their cars in another way—as vehicles to express their aggression? How, indeed, can men's aggression be contained so that it injures neither others nor themselves?

Questions like these, in the province of psychology and sociology, as well as the economic and ethical ones raised earlier, are relevant to medicine now and are likely to mount in importance. They have at present no agreed answers. To pose them at all—and this limited list omits scores of others as germane—and to suggest that they are becoming major preoccupations of medicine shows how far medicine has travelled in this century and how exciting its future is likely to be. As scientists and humanists doctors will be needed to help to provide the answers, a task—to return to George Eliot—that will certainly "call forth the highest intellectual strain".

Index